Grandmother's Wisdom Returns

The stress and strain of daily life leaves us all vulnerable to "dis-ease" in any of its many manifestations. So we run to the pharmacy counter for a quick fix of antacids, antihistamines, laxatives. We reach for the coffee pot to give us energy, for a glass of wine to calm us down. Much of what we consider to be "healing" only stresses our bodies further in the long run, while adding a strain on our pocketbooks.

Why complicate life more when there are hundreds of simple solutions—natural, time-tested solutions that cost a mere fraction of over-the-counter remedies? What worked for great- grandpa can work for you today. Got a stomachache? Try brown sugar or a raw carrot. A stuffy nose? Try garlic, apple cider vinegar or pack your feet in ice cubes. Relax with a cup of lettuce tea, relieve menstrual cramps with red raspberry juice, ease sore muscles with buttermilk, banish dandruff with parsley. These home remedies may sound crazy but they work!

Jude's Herbal Home Remedies gives you more than you could ever imagine. Along with remedies to make you feel better, you'll find recipes for quick maple syrup, chickweed pancakes, corn coffee from the Iroquois, and much more. You'll find easy home-care hints that include a natural ant repellent that won't harm pets and an amazing way to clean wallpaper with white bread! There are even intriguing activities for children. Snowed in? Make homemade fingerpaints and keep them occupied for hours.

There is beauty and majesty in natural simplicity, and here are more than 800 ways to simplify your life. Many of the ingredients required already await in your own kitchen cabinet! Others can be found in your supermarket, local health food store, or through mail order companies listed in the back of the book.

This is one book that won't collect dust on the shelf. In fact, there's probably a remedy in here that you'll want to try right now!

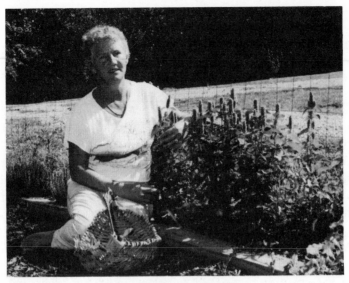

About the Author

JUDE WILLIAMS lives near Eaton Ohio. She has always been close to nature. She uses every opportunity to spread the word on the importance of learning to live in harmony with our living earth. She believes the growing interest in simple living will guide us to work with nature so that healing for ourselves and our earth can take place.

Her involvement with herbs spans 25 years. As a Master Herbalist with her degree from Dominion Herbal College, she is in demand for lectures and frequently is a guest on radio shows, discussing the topic of herbal medicine.

She divides her free time between family, grandchildren, and long walks in the woodlands, in search of wild herbs.

To Write to the Author

We cannot guarantee that every letter written to the author can be answered, but all will be forwarded. Both the author and the publisher appreciate hearing from readers, learning of your enjoyment and benefit from this book. Llewellyn also publishes a monthly news magazine with news and reviews of practical esoteric studies and articles helpful to the student. Some readers' questions and comments to the author may be answered through this magazine's columns if permission to do is included in the original letter. The author sometimes participates in seminars and workshops, and dates and places are announced in *The Llewellyn New Times*. To write to the author, or to ask a question write to:

Jude C. Williams
c/o THE LLEWELLYN NEW TIMES
P.O. Box 64383-869, St. Paul, MN 55164-0383, U.S.A.

Please enclose a self-addressed, stamped envelope for reply, or $1.00 to cover costs.

Llewellyn's Living With Nature Series

Jude's Herbal Home Remedies

Natural Health, Beauty & Home-Care Secrets

Jude C. Williams, Master Herbalist

1992
Llewellyn Publications
St. Paul, Minnesota 55164-0383, U.S.A.

FIRST EDITION, 1992
Second Printing, 1992

Cover Design by Terry Buske

Library of Congress Cataloging-in-Publication Data
Williams, Jude.
   Jude's herbal home remedies: natural health, beauty & home-care
secrets / Jude Williams.
     p.   ca. — (Living with nature series)
Includes index.
ISBN 0-87542-869-X
1. Herbs—Therapeutic use. 2. Herbal cosmetics. I. Title.
II. Title: Herbal home remedies.   III. Series.
RM666.H33W58   1992
615' .321—dc20   92-58
                                                      CIP

Llewellyn Publications
A Division of Llewellyn Worldwide, Ltd.
P.O. Box 64383, St. Paul, MN 55164-0383

    Printed on recycled paper.

Llewellyn's Living With Nature Series

It's pitch black outside, but the alarm rings anyway and we arise. We throw on a light switch so we can see to plug in the machine which pours forth the magical elixir that will keep us awake. We go out of doors just long enough to get to the car, and we fire up the engine to propel us to another building where we will sit under artificial lights and breath recirculated air. We return home nine to ten hours later, but not before stopping at yet another building with artificial lighting where we purchase our dinner in a plastic bag inside a cardboard box. And then, if we are lucky and can afford the time, we take a walk across the concrete that encircles our neighborhood. Returning to our house, we sit down in front of an electronic box to observe other people going about life in their buildings and their cars.

In the average day, the average person has little contact with "nature." Civilization as we know it has designed it that way, so that the ever-changing cycles of the days and seasons don't get in the way of our day-to-day activities. In essence, we have disassociated ourselves from the very source of ourselves: Mother Earth.

But Nature's rhythms pulse on, even when we aren't listening. Hers is the pulse of life, of health, of energy and of wholeness. It's the pulse of our inner being, our love and our passion. Ignore the pulse, and we ignore what life is all about.

Llewellyn's Living with Nature Series gives you a direct opportunity to experience the power and majesty of the natural way. The books in this series will help you tap into the life-force directly, through simple activities that are in balance with Nature. You will learn how to bring the miraculous energies of our Earth into your everyday life. And while you may not be able to change your lifestyle completely, you will begin to experience life as She designed it; as a result, you will become more balanced and complete within yourself.

Dedication

**BE STILL, AND KNOW THAT I AM GOD.
PSALMS 46:10**

I have dedicated this book with many thanks to my parents, Erbie and Hilda Todd. Without their love and teaching I would not have the interests that I now have. I was taught a great love of reading and a curiosity about life that came directly from their love and caring. I would also like to thank my husband, Carl, for his dedication to our life together. We have learned a lot together over the last thirty-two years. He has had a lot of patience, which was necessary in putting up with some of my eccentricities. He always encouraged me in whatever I attempted. My children deserve thanks also, for they were of great encouragement to me. And I would not want to forget the many friends that I have had over the years who helped me with learning about the lifestyle I love.

I also want to include a poem that my namesake, my granddaughter gave to me. I think that she shares my love of nature.

I SAW A BIRD
I SAW A TREE
I SAW THE GRASS
AND ME.

NOTICE

This book is no substitute for proper medical care. It is not intended to be a medical guide. Consult your doctor for any serious health problems.

Herbs can be very potent and must be used responsibly. Some of them can be poisonous. You are responsible for your health. The publisher assumes no responsibility for the efficacy of these recipes, nor do we promise any cures. Use caution and common sense with the recipes found in this book. Many people are allergic to some plants, so do a skin patch test before using an herb in a recipe, to test for an allergic response.

Contents

Introduction

A friend once asked me why I was so interested in the use of herbs. The answer came back before I even thought about it: the lifestyle. I got to thinking about that answer and thought, yes, that is what is so interesting about herbs. Once you get curious about the use of herbs, you get into so many different subjects that you never lose interest. The use of herbs got me to thinking about the way we live our lives.

I really became interested in herbs about 25 years ago and only recently got to study them more formally. I received my Chartered Herbalist degree from Dominion Herbal College in 1990. (Editor's note: She now has her Master Herbalist degree.) Even after these many years, herbs still hold a fascination for me. Just to think that one seed can feed a family still fills me with wonder. One plant can help to balance your system so that health can return. Stop and think about how we have lost some knowledge that should be saved and used by future generations.

I used to think I would love to live a completely natural lifestyle. Over the years I realized that the modern conveniences were given to us by our Maker to make our lives easier. We can and should combine the old with the new for our comfort. We simply have to learn how best to utilize the new, so that we don't destroy our earth by living in a throwaway society.

We have caused our young people to lose pride in their heritages by throwing out that which has brought humankind to where it is today. Now we have an obligation to let them know that what their cultures contributed is worth saving. I suppose that I am talking mostly about the young Afro-Americans and the American Indian youth in particular. Their cultures have contributed so much that we must get them to realize what they still have to offer, and encourage them to take pride in who they are.

Herbs got me to thinking about the insects that are in nature. They, too, have a part to play in the food chain. We must stop using pesticides because they are destroying the insects along with us. We have a chance to help our young people start thinking of ways to live that are more in balance with nature—otherwise we will not survive. We must start recycling everything we use in order to save our natural environment.

I really feel that you become more spiritual when you become acquainted with nature. I feel that this old world could handle that right now, don't you?

My husband and I became aware of how much our society was becoming a nation of consumers thirty years ago. That's when we decided to change our lifestyle to be more in tune with nature. We have benefited much from that decision. The more we became independent and knowledgeable about doing things for ourselves, the more we enjoyed it. We grow and can all our own fruits and vegetables. We built our own home last year and take a great deal of pride in that. Soon we will be able to provide our own electricity.

Everyday you can pick up a newspaper or magazine and read how more and more people are coming to realize that quality of life is more important than making a lot of money and more people are dropping out of the so-called fast lane. All I can say is hooray for them. They are finding out that the new lifestyle they are choosing to lead now has great benefits for their children. They are finding that they receive a great deal of satisfaction and pride in being able to do for themselves. Nothing you learn is ever wasted.

Suppose the world does have a natural or manmade catastrophe. Would you have the knowledge to provide for your family? We appreciate the modern conveniences, but we would be perfectly willing and able to live with a lot less and get a lot of pleasure doing it. I don't advocate giving up convenience for natural living. We can have the best from the past and present—and perhaps the future. The way the world is going we had best have some expertise in coping with the unknown future.

I gave serious thought to becoming a vegetarian. But, after watching the natural chain of events, and through different experiences that I have had, I came to realize that the animals are part of the food chain. They are more aware of this than humans are. Neither me nor my husband are hunters. If it came down to me having to butcher an animal in order to eat, I could be a vegetarian with no problem. But I do feel that if you need to hunt to feed your family there is nothing wrong with hunting. The wrong comes in when it is done for sport. I really feel that we should give thanks for any animal that gives its life in order to feed us and our children.

I feel that nature has a lot to teach us about beauty and attraction.The natural order of life is procreation and the attraction must be there in order to procreate. When we learn to go with the flow and become much more natural in our attitudes toward attracting the opposite sex, this helps us to stop playing all the mind games that go on with the mating game now. We soon take a more spiritual attitude toward the opposite sex, and toward relationships.

Nature teaches us about seasons. This can be related to our life changes and how everything has it's season or time for being. We learn about order from nature. Why can't we bring that order into our life? Everyday living becomes easier if there is order in our life. Even gardening is easier if we learn to work with nature instead of trying to control our environment.

So don't ask me what herbs have to offer, because I guess that I could point out just about any lifestyle that could benefit from learning even a little about our wild gifts.

I really do hope that you find something of value to use from this book. Even if you do not use the recipes, maybe it will start you thinking about how important saving our environment is for the future of humankind.

Most of our modern medicines are derived from the wild herbs, so we can at least learn to respect them in their native habitat by protecting our land and forests. We can help save the forests by recycling what we do use. We can start making our lives simpler and rediscover the values that are important to us in order to be happy. We can learn to have respect for the animals and insects that make life possible for us. We can learn to share our time and hobbies with our families and bring our families closer again. Our value system will change again. Let's hope it uses some of the old values while improving upon them with the new.

·1·

General Principles of Herbs

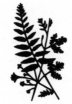

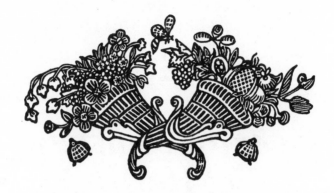

L earning to use herbs for yourself and your family's good is a lifelong process. Becoming interested in herbs is a learning process that will keep you interested for the rest of your life. It can be rewarding to be able to treat some of your family's illnesses and to learn a preventive way of living. Prevention should be the first thing that you look at when learning to keep you or your family healthy.

Because there are some illnesses that you are not able to prevent, it is good to have a family physician that you can turn to when it becomes necessary. Herbs are not meant to take the place of your family doctor; they are for simple illnesses that you would be able to treat at home.

There are also times in our lives when medical care is not available and we have to deal with certain diseases on our own. By practicing a preventive lifestyle, you will find your family has to cope with less sickness.

Often, we need to learn how to handle an emergency situation when our physician is not available. Unfortunately, many of us have also learned to seek a doctor every time we have an upset stomach or a slight cold. We are placing an unfair burden on the medical doctors and hospitals and pricing ourselves right out of medical insurance. We take prescription drugs and keep our systems full of drugs that are totally unnecessary. We would be able to respond more readily to emergency treatment if we learned to care for simple illnesses by a more natural method.

Herbs are a natural way to treat many such illnesses. Most herbs taken for treatment will pass harmlessly through the system if not needed by the body. Can you say the same for many prescriptions? Many of the prescribed drugs are stored in the liver or other organs and eventually our bodies will stop responding to a certain drug that could be a life-saver if used for emergency treatment only.

A healthy, chemical-free diet and lifestyle helps strengthen your immune system and thus allows the body to heal naturally. Also, by keeping the system chemical-free, your body reacts much more quickly and positively to any emergency treatment that your doctor may deem necessary. This means the treatment time will probably be shorter.

Learning to prepare your own herbal remedies involves much more than mixing together herbs. You must become familiar with the properties of the herbs in order to treat an illness successfully. The easiest way to become familiar with the properties of the herbs is to grow them. If you have decided to use herbal remedies, then you must decide which herbs to grow.

Long ago, most of the herbalists and shamans concentrated on just a few herbs and learned all there was to know about those. This is just about the best advice I can give you. If you try to learn about too many at once, you will waste much time. Most of the herbs serve more than one purpose and are useful for more than one remedy. Even if you purchase most of your herbs, you still have to get acquainted with the reasons for using one particular herb over another and even substituting one herb for another.

SIGNATURES OF HERBS

Many of the herbs have what are called signatures. It is important to understand what those signatures are in order to know what the herb can be used for. "Signatures" are a system of characteristics which help identify the herb and its functions. You will become proficient in gathering wild herbs once you have an understanding of the signature of the plants. (I want to mention here that with knowledge comes responsibility. Many of the wild herbs are on the endangered list, so be aware when you do use nature's bounty).

Knowing the signatures of the plants will also help you in preparing and creating your own recipes. Certain characteristics can be broken down into categories. These categories would indicate what a particular plant could be used for. Here are some general rules to help you understand signatures.

1. The color of the herb's flowers is an important part of the signature. The plants with the yellow blooms are generally used for liver, gallbladder, and all urinary problems and tonics that rid the body of toxins and infections.

The herbs with the reddish flowers are all good **blood purifiers** and/or **alteratives**. (Editor's note: See glossary for definitions of terms.) The color red indicates the **astringency** or the healing effect of certain herbs. Herbs with this color can be used to treat skin disorders that are caused by blood impurities. The active ingredient of many of the **alterative** herbs are considered to be **antibiotic** in nature.

Herbs that have purple or blue blooms are without exception used as a **sedative** or **relaxant**. These are good to add to a recipe when the patient needs to stay calm during an illness, or in treating muscle spasms. Most of our illnesses are caused by stress and most of the herbal remedies would benefit from the addition of a **calmative** or sedative. They are also considered good blood purifiers, so they would have their place in tonics as well.

2. The growing conditions of the herb would be the second thing you would look at to ascertain the signature of the herb. Herbs that grow in an area with a lot of gravel would indicate that the plant would be used in treating illnesses that have to do with stone or gravel in the body. These herbs help to cleanse and remove harmful accumulations from the **alimentary** and **bronchial** systems. They would be used to treat kidney stones or gallstones.

So-called stone-breakers are parsley, peppergrass, shepherd's purse, sassafras and mullein. Mullein will grow just about anywhere. I find it quite often growing in gravel along railways and roadways.

You would not necessarily use the same kind of plants or herbs if you found them growing in other conditions. For instance, milkweed growing in sandy soil has twice as many active ingredients as the same species found growing in a good, rich soil.

Herbs found growing in mucky, swampy, or wet ground are good to use in recipes designed to treat excessive **mucous excretions**, such as respiratory problems dealing with asthma, colds, coughs, and rheumatic disorders. Willow, verbena, boneset, and elder are examples of this.

Herbs that grow near fast-moving water are good to use as **diuretics**. These help to clean the **alimentary** systems of toxins and harmful wastes.

Always be aware of the growing conditions when gathering herbs for a specific treatment. A good example of differences found in the herbs is the sage plant. Sometimes a pink and a blue bloom will be found on the same species of sage growing right next to each other. This would indicate to me that the blue-flowered plant would be used only as a **sedative**. Because of the **astringent** nature of sage, both pink and blue-flowered sage could be used as a blood purifier, but I would choose the pink-blossomed plant, because the pink flowers would indicate that it has more blood purifying properties.

3. Different textures indicate different uses. Herbs that have a soft texture to them would be useful for treating swollen or inflamed areas. They would also be used in so-called wet colds or any chest disorders. No herbal remedy for internal use would be considered complete unless one of these **emollient** herbs is included in the recipe. Horehound, mullein and hollyhocks are good examples of emollient herbs.

4. Any of the herbs that have thorns or are prickly are used in disorders where there is sharp pain. Thistle is used as a tonic for all the organs. Hawthorn can be used as a tonic for the heart because it has sharp thorns and is indicative of sharp pains in the heart. Hawthorn is also considered a diuretic and that would be helpful in any heart treatment. Wild prickly lettuce is used as a pain reliever and as a sedative. It has blossoms that may be white, yellow or blue. The prickles are indicative of its usefulness in treating sharp pain.

The **epidermal** hairs of some of the plants are suggestive of their use in internal problems where there are sharp pains, or a stitching pain. Hops, nettle, and mullein are three plants that come to mind immediately.

5. Any herb that clings to itself is believed to cling to, and help remove any hardened mucus of the inner systems. Any of the

herbs that have a "sticking to" propensity are good to use in ridding the body of toxins and virus germs. Balm of Gilead is used in chest complaints because it has a sticky substance covering it. The ground-covering herbs are also considered good to use in ridding the body of hardened mucus. Examples of this are coltsfoot, sage, thyme, horehound and mallow.

6. Herbs that are also vines are considered good to use in remedies for the blood system and the nervous system because they resemble them. The blood vessels and the nerve paths throughout the body call to mind the vines. Another way to check whether or not the herb would be useful for these disorders is to check the root system of the plant. If it has a vein-like root system, then the herb could be used to treat disorders dealing with the blood system or nervous disorders. Even if the herb is not a vine, the root system would be indicative of use in those areas.

7. The skin healers have signatures in several different ways. They have thin, threadlike roots and stems. Cinquefoil, gold thread and septfoil are good examples of this. The roots resemble the structure of the veins in the skin.

8. Fissures in the bark of certain trees would be indicative of their use in certain skin disorders. Cherry, white birch, and elder are examples of trees with healing properties for skin ulcers and sores. Balsamic resinous exudations help to heal cuts and ulcers of the skin. Moss, lichens and molds are good choices when making preparations used to treat skin diseases (such as psoriasis) because these herbs resemble the appearance of these disorders.

9. Sometimes, just the name alone can indicate the use of that particular herb. Heartsease, eyebright, pleurisy root, feverfew, cancer root, and throat root are just a few. Many of the plants, such as eyebright and chamomile, are indicative for eyes because the floral parts resemble eyes.

10. Many of the herbs that have a root structure resembling the human torso are used as aphrodisiacs, or as a way to overcome sterility. Ginseng is an example of this.

Skullcap and walnut have forms that resemble the shape of the human head, and can be used in treatment of headaches and nervous disorders.

11. Another important herbal signature is aroma. The strong-smelling herbs such as cinnamon, cloves, thyme and rosemary are used as disinfectants. Most of the aromatic herbs are highly **antiseptic** or **germicidal** and have **antibiotic** properties. Sage, pennyroyal, all mints, tansy and yarrow are good examples.

12. Another good rule to remember: herbs which attract bees can also be used as an antidote for bee and insect bites. Bee balm and basil are good examples of this. Just crush several leaves and rub on the area.

Some of the signatures will not apply in every case. There are some herbs that have no signature. Study the properties of the plant that you plan to use and become familiar with the signature of that plant (or lack of signature) before using it in any recipe.

Becoming familiar with the signatures of the the herbs is a first step in getting control over our health. When the ancient shamans and healers concentrated on just a few plants and became experts in the use of those few, their remedies were effective. Diet played an important part in their treatments. They realized that a healthy diet was linked to a healthy body and a healthy mind.

We live in a world that has become dangerous to our health and we should start where we can do the most good. Taking care of those we love and teaching them to take care of their body, spirit, and mind is the most important difference we can make. By studying about the ways Mother Nature can make our life better, we also become more spiritually-minded. We soon realize that we are all connected and learn ways to deal with our own excesses. We learn to work with nature and not against it. We learn that we are responsible for our own health and take steps to keep healthy.

HERBAL HISTORY

If we are to become knowledgeable about herbs we should have a little history about them. Herbs have always contributed to human health. Their use goes far back into antiquity. One of the first well-known and important books written about herbs is attributed to a Greek physician, Dioscorides. *De Materis Medica* (the title in Latin) was written about A.D. 60. The manuscript was used as a reference source by many herbalists. It was circulated for hundreds of years throughout the Middle East and the West. It contained the properties of over 600 plants.

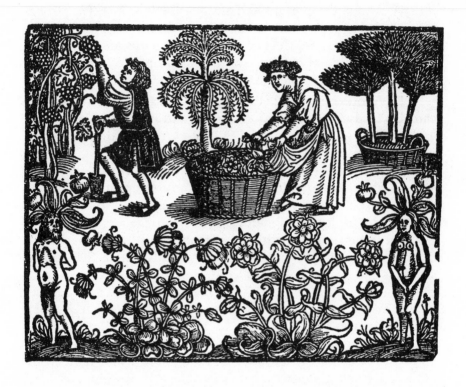

Occasionally, superstition became associated with the use of herbs, but basically the information was founded on sound plant lore and use. Ancient herbalists became familiar with the uses of the herbs through experience. The knowledge was kept and handed down through the ages by people like you and me.

Documents found in the ancient pyramids were passed on to the Greeks, then to the Romans. Many different sources comment on the uses of herbs. Herbs are mentioned in the Bible as well as many of the sacred books of our major religions. The Druids were among the first known to use the plants in religious rites.

In Great Britain, monasteries served as early herbal laboratories. The Monks grew, collected and used the herbs. They kept records of their uses. They opened hospitals and were among the first to use the plants in a scientific way. Their herbal knowledge soon became commonplace. Today, we have reached the point where we can again, with increased appreciation, learn to use these natural products.

Many people still think that learning to use herbs is too complex, too involved, so they don't even try to become knowledgeable about how to use them. If they only knew how big a part herbs play in their lives right now. Every tree, shrub, flower and plant is an herb, and I believe that they are all useful. We just don't know what all the uses are right now.

Modern scientists are studying the uses of herbs; we are getting new products and medicines every day. Herbalists have long known what can be used because that information was passed down to them. Now we will be able to prove or disprove some of the folklore surrounding the herbs. Most of the old herbal remedies are proving to be valid and are used today in modern medicines. Digitalin, found in foxglove, is still in use today to treat heart disorders. At least 75% of all prescribed medications come from the herbs. Even the spices we use daily have their part to play in modern medical uses.

Throughout history, people have been healed by using herbal extracts that were not in common use by the medical profession of their time. Some of these spices are still used today by pharmacologists in preparing prescribed medications. They are finding that many of the old herbal remedies have fewer side effects and are effective in helping to balance the body's system. Researchers have found, for example, that milk thistle (*Cardnus marianus*) does contain properties that carry bile from the liver. It was used for centuries for this purpose before modern scientists tested the plant. They found that it does stimulate regenerative growth of liver cells, promoting self-repair in a damaged liver. It is used in treatment of hepatitis and cirrhosis of the liver.

Mint is an example of an old favorite that is used in new ways. It is used extensively for many of our products. We use it in gums, candies, teas, toothpaste, mouthwashes, and as a flavoring or in prescribed medications. It is now a cash crop that yields 50 pounds of oil per acre.

We have learned much about herbs from the American Indians. They taught the first English settlers how to use many different herbs. Milkweed is still used today to treat poison ivy, ringworm, and a host of other skin ailments. It is also considered to be a food. Early American physicians used the root to treat asth-

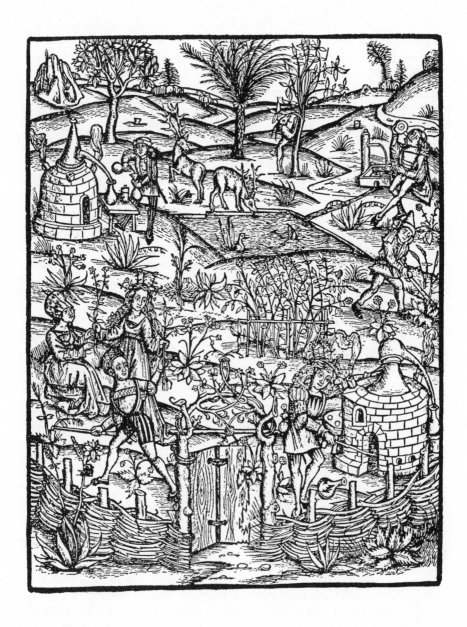

A Mediaeval Garden of Herbs from Brunschwig's LIBER DE ARTE DISTILLANDI, *Strassburg, Grüninger, 1500*

ma and other respiratory problems. The down was used to stuff life jackets during World War II. Because the milkweed down has insulating properties, it has been and is still in use today as stuffing for jackets, pillows, and blankets. How much more can be expected from a single plant? It fed us, clothed us, and served as a medicinal remedy—yet few people give the common milkweed any credit for being so useful. It is sprayed, cut down and destroyed wherever it is found.

The same can be said of cattail. The roots of cattails serve as a food, the pods are crushed and used to insulate jackets, blankets and such. It serves to insulate, as well as being waterproof. The leaves are used to make baskets, and serve other purposes as well. So, what do we do, we cut it down, spray it, and destroy a natural resource. However, we still use the pods to enhance fall bouquets and flower arrangements.

Another herb with many uses is tarragon. It is used extensively for food enhancement now, but in ancient times it was called Dragon Herb because it was used as an antidote for treating the bites of venomous animals. About 1650, tarragon was transported to America where it was used to induce menstruation. As a poultice, it is still used to treat bruises and swellings.

Red clover tea is still in use today to treat colds, fevers and debilitating diseases. The Native Americans used red clover in a salve to treat burns. It was also used as a pot herb. A pot herb is a green, leafy vegetable, often served as a side dish for meals. Red clover is a member of the pea family and has many of the same crucial vitamins and minerals. We should take advantage of that fact by using the plant.

Native Americans also used raspberry root bark to treat many illnesses. Pharmacologists today admit that there is value in using the tea for childbirth and painful menstruation because it does contain a substance that helps one to relax, as well as a stimulant for the uterine muscles.

I must admit that I have an ulterior motive for getting you interested in using herbs. I feel that as you become more aware of the uses of the herbs, you will develop a respect for Mother Nature. If herbs become important to you, you would probably become more protective of our environment and start to practice habits that save our natural resources and gifts. As you become more aware of our environment, you practice better health habits and this leads to a more spiritual lifestyle. This in turn makes you even more aware of your responsibilities to Mother Earth in a spiritual way.

We all have own paths to take through life. Edgar Cayce said, "First the individual, then to the group, then to the classes, then to the masses." And that's where it all starts. Once we become aware, we teach by example. No one person is exempt from this responsibility. If we are to save our planet, we must start now by taking an interest in nature, in our surroundings.

We have many prophets telling us that the time will come when we have no choices left. I feel that we are on that threshold now. We have no more time to waste. We must all start where we are now, to help in some way to make a difference. By taking a step, even a small step in the right direction, doors will open that will amaze you. When the student is ready, the teacher appears. There are many teachers out there, we just have to learn how to listen. Really we are all teachers, because a person does make a difference with each and every action. Every person you meet will be affected by your practices, beliefs and actions. Example is and always has been the best teacher. Many of the visionaries of our time are calling out to us, loud and clear. We have to learn to listen. Will we?

Edgar Cayce, the sleeping prophet, said we must become nature-based if we are to survive. Sun Bear, another great prophet of our time, has devoted his life to advocating a simpler lifestyle, one that is nature-based.

A simpler life style does not mean giving up modern conveniences; we must simply learn to use them wisely. Edgar Cayce said that our weaknesses could become our strengths, if we knew how to direct those weaknesses. Stubbornness could be transformed into a quality that makes for leadership; anger and hostility could become courage and boldness; deception could become inventiveness; sensuality could lead to healing. If we simply learn to redirect our energies, a bad habit becomes a blessing for ourselves, as well as for those around us. We learn to relate our beliefs to our everyday life.

By studying our pathway today, we discover hidden talents. Consider your interests, talents and hobbies. This will lead you in the correct direction on your path. Talents express the creative energy of each soul. These are to be used, not wasted.

More and more we are becoming aware of the delicate balance on this planet of ours, and we can give thanks to the people that have dedicated their lives to changing prevailing views. So in my small way, I want to introduce you to herbs with the hope that this will help you on your earth walk. Just keep in mind that for every plant, there is a use. Maybe you will be the one to discover just what that use is as you become more interested in what nature has to offer.

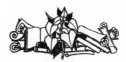

What better way to get acquainted with herbs and Mother Nature than to grow your own herbs. To begin your herb bed, start with the space you have available. You may be surprized at how much space you have to devote to a useful bed of herbs. Many people think that herbs are not attractive, yet they are unaware of the attractive herbs already growing in their flower beds. Bee balm, calendula, roses, barberry, feverfew and hollyhocks are just a few that come to mind.

There are many different designs to use when planning your herb bed. The major factor is space. The more formal gardens naturally need more room. If this design appeals to you, you may have to sacrifice some of your yard to your herb beds. Many people plan on using their whole yard as an attractive herb garden. Creating paths and special places to sit make the garden enjoyable to all.

If you want a large garden, your plan should be to take several years so that the project does not become so overpowering and so expensive that you lose interest and give up. Gathering the rocks for your pathways can be a project that your whole family can be involved with. The more natural the items that you use to create your garden, the more beautiful the finished project.

Part of my interest in herbs comes from my desire to become more natural in my lifestyle. This does include saving money. You would be surprised at how creative you become when you set a money limit on your materials. Another way to save money is to trade herb starts with other herbalists. Or, if you are successful in starting the herb plants and have the time needed to care for many small plants, you could start the plants and sell them to make your garden pay for itself.

The patterns you can use to create your beds are endless. Study some of the books on garden design to find the one that suits you and your lifestyle. It is good to give some thought to what you want to put in your garden. Once in, it is more difficult

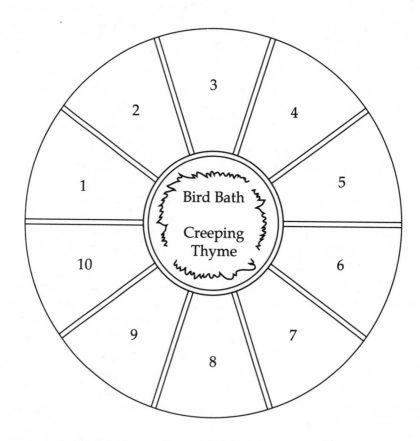

Simple Wheel Design

1	Holy basil	6	Lemon balm
2	Tansy	7	Mint
3	Comfrey	8	Roman chamomile
4	Eyebright	9	Thyme
5	Bee balm	10	Sage

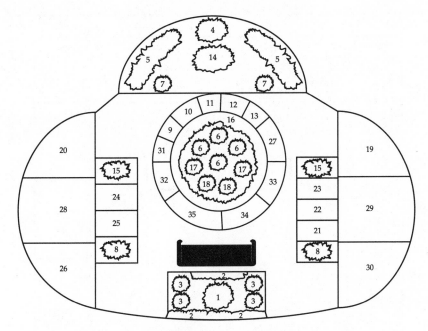

English Country Garden

1 Crab apple tree	10 German chamomile	19 Elderberry	28 Mint
2 Mother-of-thyme	11 Holy basil	20 Hyssop	29 Horehound
3 Sweet woodruff	12 Comfrey	21 Chives	30 Coriander
4 Willow	13 Dill	22 Garlic chives	31 Garlic
5 Red raspberries	14 Soapwort	23 Oregano	32 Lemon balm
6 White roses	15 Costmary	24 Parsley	33 Lemon thyme
7 Hollyhocks	16 Pennyroyal	25 Feverfew	34 Lemon-scented
8 Broom	17 Violet	26 Anise hyssop	marigold
9 White yarrow	18 Nasturtium	27 Sage	35 Basil

to make changes and may cost you a growing season of using your herbs.

Once you have decided which kinds of herbs to plant, look at the growing habits of the herbs selected. You may want to contain a few in the corners of your yard to keep them from taking over your beds. I am thinking in particular of the mints, as they are so sociable that they like to visit all the other herbs, and sometimes move in with them permanently.

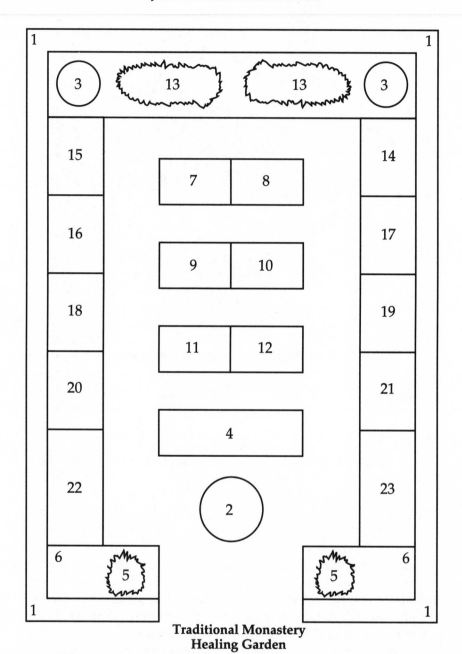

**Traditional Monastery
Healing Garden**

1 Yew hedge	5 Broom	9 Eyebright	13 Roses	17 Yarrow	21 Anise
2 Crab apple tree	6 Lavender	10 Horehound	14 Costmary	18 Lemon balm	22 Sage
3 Honeysuckle	7 Soapwort	11 St. John's wort	15 Coriander	19 Mint	23 Chamomile
4 Sweet woodruff	8 Bee balm	12 Feverfew	16 Rue	20 Lamb's ears	

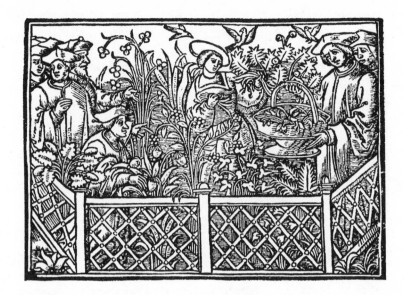

I have a particular love of the wild herbs, and fortunately I live surrounded by woods. I am planting and transplanting some of the wild herbs throughout the woods. This week I need to transplant some of the jewelweed because they are growing where we are placing an acre pond. While prowling around looking for a good place to move them, I also found some Solomon's Seal that I will try to transplant.

I have fought tooth and nail to save a blackberry patch. And I won! The drive to the pond will be moved and my berries are saved. The wild yarrow will also have to be moved as they are growing right where the path to the proposed barn is. I guess this will be a never-ending project for me and I'm going to love every minute of it.

Because there are so many different herbs, you may want to concentrate on just a few species. There are so many different flavors in some of the species that you may want to concentrate on just one species, perhaps a bed filled with many varieties of thyme.

There is a saying that when in doubt, use thyme, as there are so many different herb flavors that can be substituted with thyme. The taste of some of the thymes can be amazingly like the taste of other herbs. To name a few, there is lemon thyme, golden thyme, English thyme, nutmeg thyme, woolly thyme, french thyme, caraway thyme and the list could go on and on. Any of the thymes can be used as an astringent in the herbal remedies. Thyme is also used in cooking, potpourri, and many hobbies. A round bed with nothing but different kinds of thyme is a very attractive sight.

If you plan on growing large quantities of herbs for home use, perhaps the easiest way would be to grow them in rows in your vegetable garden. Some of the herbs that you use frequently could be planted close to your kitchen door for ease of gathering. If you plan to create a bee colony, there are special herbs to plant near your hives. Some herbs act as a natural herbicide if planted as companion plants for those plants that you wish to protect. Just determine what your needs are and go from there.

It is always good to learn the properties of the herbs as you plant them. This may take more time in getting an established bed, but it is well worth the effort. If you educate yourself about some ways to use each plant, you know you will get full use of your herb garden. As you come to understand that one plant can be used in many different remedies, you may find that a large herb garden is unnecessary.

If you plan on using wild herbs only, please become aware of the plants that are on our endangered list and learn to conserve and save our natural resources. Ginseng was almost totally destroyed early in this century by people who gathered the herb to sell. It was literally worth it's weight in gold and was much in demand worldwide. Even Daniel Boone gathered it to sell because it was more profitable than hunting or trapping.

By ordering wild herbs to plant, you will learn to identify the plants and learn about their growing needs, too. This is very important when first learning to use the plants for remedies. Never gather wild herbs without being absolutely positive of the identification of the plants. It is a good idea to use several different reference books to help you learn to identify the herbs.

When planting your herbs, be aware of the plant's needs. You would not plant an herb that needs a shady area if you can provide no shade. Once you have decided what herbs are important for you to cultivate, it becomes much easier to plan your garden. This list should help you to get started. I've included the height of the plants so you can place the taller herbs in the back of the bed. I recommend that you draw a garden plan before you start planting. Drawing a plan is easy and will save you much effort later on. This list includes some of the more common herbs that you would probably use in making herbal home remedies.

ALOE VERA *(Aloe spp.)*: One to two feet tall. Grow in pots for indoor use. Good to treat burns and skin disorders.

ANGELICA *(Angelica archangelica)*: Five to eight feet tall. Use in remedies to treat digestive and bronchial problems. *Caution:* It may make you more sensitive to the sun and is potentially toxic.

ANISE *(Pimpinella anisum)*: Two feet tall. Used to treat gastric problems and to increase milk production in nursing mothers.

ARNICA *(Arnica montana)*: One to two feet tall. Liniments and salves are made from arnica. *Caution:* Not for internal use.

BASIL *(Ocimum basilicum)*: One to two feet tall. Use it to treat digestive problems and have handy to rub on bee stings to prevent swelling and pain.

BAY LEAF *(Laurus nobilis)*: Plant in pot for indoor cultivation. Good for indigestion.

BEE BALM *(Monarda didyma)*: Three to four feet tall. Use for colds, fevers, coughs, nausea, indigestion and menstrual cramps.

BETONY *(Stachys officinalis)*: Three feet tall. Use for asthma, bronchitis, heartburn and kidney problems. Juice is used to heal cuts; make a poultice for sprains.

BIRCH *(Betula spp.)*: Black birch leaves relieve headaches and rheumatism, fevers, kidney stones, and cramps. They also make a pleasant-tasting beer.

BONESET (*Eupatorium perfoliatum*): Two to five feet tall. Added to teas and remedies to treat colds, aches and pains associated with flu symptoms.

BORAGE (*Borago officinalis*): Two to three feet tall. Relieves depression; treats fevers and bronchitis. Poultices made from the leaves reduce swelling and pain. *Caution:* It may cause dermatitus in sensitive people. Prolonged use is not advised.

CALENDULA (*Calendula officinalis*): One to two feet tall. Great to treat ulcers of the leg associated with varicose veins. Great salve for cuts and bruises. This herb is a must to plant.

CARDAMOM (*Elettaria cardamomum*): Six to twelve feet tall. Chew seeds to relieve flatulence and ease indigestion. Natural breath sweetener. Usually grows in the tropics.

CAYENNE PEPPER (*Capsicum annuum*): Approximately one foot tall. Several plants will provide plenty of peppers. Good for treating everything from high blood pressure to stomach ulcers. Good tonic for the heart and blood system.

CHAMOMILE (*Chamaemelum nobile* and *Matricaria recutita*): Two to three feet tall. Relaxes, so it can be used for everything from reducing depression to sleep disorders. Also relieves headaches.

CHERVIL (*Anthriscus cerefolium*): About two feet tall. Considered a diuretic, an expectorant and a stimulant. Lowers high blood pressure, and you can use it as a wash for skin disorders.

CHICORY (*Cichorium intybus*): Three to five feet tall. Root tea is a good tonic. Tea from flowers are a great sedative and are used to treat nervous disorders.

CHIVES (*Allium schoenoprasum*): One to one and a half feet tall. Lowers blood pressure.

CLARY SAGE (*Salvia sclarea*): Three to four feet tall. Leaves are used to heal wounds, sores, insect bites and as a tonic for colic or intestinal upsets. Use as a mouth wash for cankers and for sore throats. Tea from seeds are used for eye wash.

COLTSFOOT (*Tussilago farfara*): Six inches tall when flowering. Great to use in cough syrups and to treat any bronchial problems.

COMFREY (*Symphytum officinale*): Three to five feet tall. Poultice made from comfrey leaves is to heal sprains. Wash made from the leaves is great to heal cuts in humans and animals. Destroys harmful bacteria. Also has pain relieving properties.

CORIANDER (*Coriandrum sativum*): Two to three feet tall. Aids digestion. Used as a flavoring in cough syrups or other medicinal mixtures.

COSTMARY (*Chrysanthemum balsamita*): Three feet tall. Also called Bible Leaf. Used to keep away silverfish. Leaves are used to make medicinal teas as a tonic for the liver, and as a diuretic. You can also use in salves for cuts and sores that are hard to heal.

DANDELION (*Taraxacum officinale*): Six inches to one foot tall. Used in tonics to treat liver disorders, diabetes, anemia. Also very useful as a diuretic.

DILL (*Anethum graveolens*): Three feet tall. Increases milk production for nursing mothers; also good for flatulence, colic and stomach disorders.

DOCK (*Rumex spp.*): One to four feet tall. Leaves applied to burns, cuts, and scrapes. It also makes an excellent tonic.

ECHINACEA (*Echinacea angustifolia*): One to two feet tall. Roots are used mainly as a blood purifier and wound healer.

ELECAMPANE (*Inula helenium*): Four to six feet tall. Roots are used in cough syrups and in any remedy to treat bronchial problems.

EYEBRIGHT (*Euphrasia officinalis*): Two to eight inches tall. Used in making eye wash. Make sure your wash is sterile if you are going to use it.

FENNEL (*Foeniculum vulgare*): Four feet tall. Treatment for gastritis, colic and increases milk production for both humans and animals.

 FENUGREEK (*Trigonella foenum-graecum*): One to two feet tall. All around medicinal purposes.

FEVERFEW (*Chrysanthemum parthenium*): Two to three feet tall. Used medicinally for fevers.

FOXGLOVE (*Digitalis purpurea*): Two to four feet tall. Grow for curiosity and looks only. Affects the heart rate and ***not to be used for home remedies*** to treat existing heart diseases. Leave that treatment to your family physician.

GARLIC (*Allium sativum*): Garlic has all around uses medicinally. In your diet, it can keep colds away and helps your heart to stay healthy.

GERMANDER (*Teucrium chamaedrys*): Two feet tall. Treats sore throats, dropsy, gout, and rheumatism. Has pain killing properties.

GINGER (*Zingiber officinale):* Six to sixteen inches tall. Treatment for vertigo, nausea, heart tonic, blood tonic, treats arthritis and is a good all around herb.

GINSENG (*Panax quinquefolius*): Six to sixteen inches. Ginseng has many uses. Great tonic for the whole body and is used as an aphrodisiac.

GOLDENROD (*Solidago spp*): Six to seven feet tall. Wound healer and diuretic. Goldenrod has many useful properties.

 GOLDENSEAL (*Hydrastis canadensis*): Six to twelve inches. Great heal-all and a good tonic.

HOPS (*Humulus lupulus*): Twenty to twenty-five feet vine. Great sedative. Hops are used to make beer.

HOLLYHOCKS (*Althea rosea*): Six feet tall. Great for chest complaints.

HOREHOUND (*Marrubium vulgare*): Two to three feet tall. Cough syrups and cough drops. Great to use for any chest or throat complaint.

HORSERADISH (*Armoracia rusticana*): Two to three feet tall in the second year of growth. Many uses medicinally.

HYSSOP (*Hyssopus officinalis*): Two to three feet tall. Hyssop is a cleansing herb. Used for colds, fevers, sore throats, and bronchitis. Licorice flavored hyssop makes a good tasting tea.

LAVENDER (*Lavandula angustifolia*): Up to three feet tall. Good to soothe nervous disorders.

LEMON BALM (*Melissa officinalis*): Two feet tall. Lemon balm is a great all around herb to have. Great wash for cuts and scrapes and you can use it as a tonic.

LEMON VERBENA (*Aloysia triphylla*): Grow indoors where it can reach heights of six feet or more. Great to bring about sweating to break colds, fevers and flu. Good tonic and good cleanser for cuts and scrapes. Make into cough drops.

LOBELIA (*Lobelia inflata*): One to three feet tall. Treat chest complaints. It should be used with great care as an overdose could be fatal.

LOVAGE (*Levisticum officinale*): Five feet tall. Regulates menstruation.

MARJORAM (*Origanum majorana*): One foot tall. Use to treat asthma, rheumatism and has many other uses.

MARSH MALLOW (*Althaea officinalis*): Four to five feet tall. Great for chest complaints. Hollyhock is often used as a substitute for marsh mallow.

MINTS (*Mentha spp.*): Two feet tall. Because there are so many different kinds of mints, taste would indicate which to plant for your own use. All the mints are considered to be astringents. Peppermint and spearmint are considered to be the most versatile.

MULLEIN (*Verbascum thapsus*): Three to six feet tall. Mullein is one of the most versatile of the herbs. Every part can be used. Great diuretic and liver tonic. Skin disorders, cuts, scrapes, and bruises are all treated with mullein. Good to use for chest complaints and asthma.

NASTURTIUM (*Tropaeolum majus*): One feet tall. Considered a stimulant. Good tea to use as a tonic. Has a nice peppery taste and can be used in salads and spreads.

NEW JERSEY TEA (*Ceanothus americanus*): Two to three feet tall. similar to Chinese green tea. Many uses. Use for respiratory problems and to treat high blood pressure.

ONION (*Allium cepa*): Many uses. If eaten regularly, helps to control blood pressure and heart problems.

OREGANO (*Origanum spp.*): One foot tall. Many uses. Olive oil and oregano mixed is a good rub for arthritis.

PANSY (*Viola tricolor*): Also called heartsease. Good for treating bronchial coughs and asthmatic complaints.

PARSLEY (*Petroselinum crispum*): One to one-half feet tall. Parsley is one of the best herbs to treat kidney complaints. Great diuretic to use during weight loss.

 PASSION FLOWER (*Passiflora incarnata*): Vine. Passion flower tea has sedative value.

PENNYROYAL (*Hedeoma pulegioides):* Four to sixteen inches. Pennyroyal is a gentle stimulant. Relieves nervous stomach. Should not be taken by pregnant women as the oil can cause uterine contraction. Good to drink during menstrual cycle.

PLANTAIN (*Plantago major*): Six to eighteen inches. Plantain is a great tonic and is used mainly for it's diuretic effect.

POPLAR (*Populus spp. salicaceae*): Ninety feet tall. The buds are gathered in the spring for use in treating chest complaints. The buds are known as balm of Gilead. Use in preparing cough syrups and for asthma complaints.

ROSE (*Rosa spp.*): Hips are great to use in preventing colds and for treating colds and the flu bug.

ROSEMARY (*Rosmarinus officinalis*): Native to the Mediterranean coast, rosemary will grow very satisfactorily in pots to be kept indoors. Rosemary can be used to treat heart palpitations if used in a cordial. It will also stimulate the urinary organs. Good for headaches and sleep disorders. *Caution:* It can be fatal in excessive amounts.

SAGE (*Salvia officinalis*): One to one and one-half feet tall. Sage is astringent in nature and can be used for everything from hair rinse to treating nervous disorders. *Caution:* It can cause symptoms of poisoning if taken in excess.

ST. JOHN'S WORT (*Hypericum perforatum*): Two feet tall. The flowers make a good ointment to use for general skin disorders. The tea is good to strengthen the immune system. Studies are being done on using St. John's Wort to fight cancer and AIDS. Can cause photo-sensitivity if used to excess.

SAVORY (*Satureja spp.*): One foot tall. Said to be an aphrodisiac. Regulates menstrual cycles and is good to treat stomach disorders.

SOAPWORT (*Saponaria officinalis*): One to two feet tall. Great to use as a natural shampoo. Also used to wash delicate items such as lace because it is very gentle.

SWEET CICELY (*Myrrhis odorata*): Three feet tall. Use to treat digestive disorders. It is considered to be an expectorant and can be used to treat colds and chest complaints. Used as a tonic for elderly people and babies.

SWEET WOODRUFF (*Galium odoratum*): Eight inches in height. Is considered a calmative, diaphoretic and a diuretic. Soothing to the stomach. Tonic for liver and heart. Also used as a base in perfumes.

TANSY (*Tanacetum vulgare*): Three to four feet tall. Tansy is an astringent, so it could be used to treat skin disorders. For external use only.

TARRAGON (*Artemisia dracunculus*): Two feet tall. Relieves many gastric disorders.

THYME (*Thymus vulgaris*): One foot tall. Great astringent. Used internally and also for external remedies. If too much is ingested, it can over-stimulate the thyroid gland and lead to poisoning.

VALERIAN (*Valeriana officinalis*): Three and one-half to five feet tall. One of the best herbs to use for home remedies. Great to use for chest complaints and is a wonderful relaxant. It should be used sparingly (only once per day) because extended use may produce poisoning. If used regularly, discontinue after 2-3 weeks.

VIOLET (*Viola odorata*): Four to six inches. Violets are a wonder plant. All parts can be used. The plant has more vitamin A than any other known plant. Great tea and a wonderful relaxant.

WILLOW (*Salix spp.*): Willow teas made from the twigs, bark and leaves are great pain relievers. Originally aspirin was made from willow bark. Now aspirin is made from petroleum and coal tar products. Can be used internally and externally to relieve pain and swelling.

YARROW (*Achillea millefolium):* Three feet tall. Has pain relieving properties similar to willow, and relieves pain when used to clean wounds and cuts. Also antiseptic in nature so it would also be used to prevent infection of wounds and cuts.

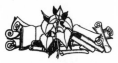

The following is a list of the herbs, placing them in categories. They will be listed as stimulants, diuretics, expectorants, astringents, nervines or sedatives. Herbs used in tonics will also be listed. You may see the same herb listed under all categories. This is because most of the herbs have more than one property and can be used in many different ways.

STIMULANTS: These herbs increase stimulus to the system and will increase blood circulation.

all mints	red clover	ginseng
calendula	ginger root	raspberry
cloves	lobelia	nettle
parsley	white yarrow	pennyroyal
balm of Gilead	caraway seed	cinnamon
anise	valerian	lemon balm
hyssop	yerba santa	cayenne pepper
coriander seed	rosemary	blue cohosh
shepherd's purse	comfrey	chervil
sage	St. John's wort	

DIURETICS: Diuretics increase the output of urine, taking harmful substances from the system.

mugwort	corn silk	burdock
plantain	pennyroyal	balm of Gilead
chamomile	dandelion	nettle
parsley	red raspberry	St. John's Wort

DIURETICS (*continued*):

shepherd's purse	carrot	thyme
water nasturtium	nasturtium	anise
or watercress	elder	garden strawberry
wild strawberry	cramp bark	borage
sage	heartsease	sweet basil
mullein	apples	comfrey
nettle	asparagus	chervil
lemon balm	savory	

EXPECTORANTS: These herbs cause the expulsion of mucus and break up congestion.

boneset	coltsfoot	anise
slippery elm	Irish moss	elecampane root
ginger	garlic	horehound
St. John's Wort	wild cherry bark	balm of Gilead
lobelia	sassafras	mullein
heartsease	prickly lettuce	comfrey
nettle	chervil	betony
comfrey	costmary	hollyhocks
marsh mallow	horseradish	hyssop
sweet cicily	bee balm	lemon balm
borage	mullein	lemon verbena
balm of Gilead		

ASTRINGENTS: Astringents are natural cleansers and are antibiotic in nature.

witch hazel	cinnamon	rosemary
thyme	comfrey	eyebright
all the mints	calendula	shepherd's purse
nettle	sage	white yarrow
plantain	bee balm	willow bark
sweet basil	chervil	garlic
hyssop	tansy	lemon balm
borage	mullein	balm of Gilead

NERVINES: Nervines relieve nervous irritation caused by strain and tension.

hops	motherwort	rosemary
chamomile	cramp bark	lettuce
red clover	valerian	violet
basil	blue cohosh	pennyroyal
skullcap	catnip	sage
passion flower	corn flowers	chicory
chervil	comfrey	rosemary
willow	lavender	borage
lobelia	yarrow	heartsease

TONICS: Tonics benefit the whole body. They strengthen the organs that are affected by the action of the digestive system. They do take time to work. So keep the treatment going until the system has time to adjust.

corn silk	burdock	white yarrow
nasturtium	sassafras	hops
dandelion	lavender	cayenne pepper
comfrey	ginger	ginseng
rosemary	all mints	anise
cinnamon	red clover	nettle
parsley	red raspberry	willow bark
chicory	shepherd's purse	costmary
goldenseal	lemon balm	mullein
heartsease	violet	

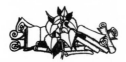

There is one small caution that I feel must be added. Most people are already aware of what they are allergic to. People have many different food allergies and this can be true of the herbs also. If you have a ragweed allergy you would know to stay away from chamomile as it is a member of the ragweed family. In some of the beauty recipes, lanolin is used. If you are allergic to lanolin, you would need to substitute olive oil or almond oil. Just be aware of your personal needs when using the herbs, eating foods, or having anything that can be used to excess to your detriment. *If you have an allergic reaction to any of the preparations, stop the treatment immediately and try another remedy.* There are so many different substitutions that you need not get discouraged. Because we are all unique, our systems will react differently to the different herbs.

Also be aware that a health problem may be caused by an allergy from common foods such as milk or wheat. Many hyperactive children are simply suffering from a common food allergy. Withholding these bothersome foods helps the child to return to natural behavior without drug treatment.

Herb preparations can safely be given to children. Small babies, ages 0 to 5 years old, should receive *one-third* the dose that an adult would receive. Children ages 5 through 12 get *one-half* of the dose that an adult would get.

Honey should never be given to children under the age of one. The American Academy of Pediatrics has placed the blame on honey for causing botulism in small children. Use sugar to sweeten any herbal mixture that you plan on using to treat small children.

Many people get the mistaken notion that if a little bit helps, a lot more is better. This is far from true. It works the same way that feeding your house plants does. You can burn your plants by adding too much commercial food the same way that you can burn the plants by adding too much manure tea. Even though manure tea is a natural way to feed your plants, *too much of a good thing can be harmful.* Just be aware of these cautions and you and your herbs will get along just fine.

·2·

Beauty Preparations

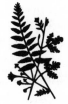

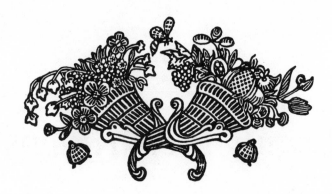

Beauty products are important to our physical and mental health. Many commercial beauty products contain artificial chemicals and these chemical substances do penetrate the skin. Every time we apply any of the commercial products to our body, we are absorbing substances through our skin that we would never dream of putting in our mouth.

By keeping well-groomed, we are also helping our self-esteem and mental health. Mental health is extremely important for physical health. By using natural products we are protecting our health.

The natural recipes are simple to make. Try different ones to find the one that works for you. Just keep in mind that if your skin has a tendency to be dry, you would not want to use too many astringents. And, keep in mind any allergies you might have. Before making any remedy, try each of the herbs in a skin test. You may not be aware of some of the allergies that you have. Each person in your family has different needs, so be aware of this as you make different recipes and preparations, recipes that members of your home will be using.

Soap can be harsh to your skin, taking away necessary natural oils, so try bathing without commercial soaps. I know it doesn't sound like very good advice, but try it for one week and see the difference for yourself. I shower most of the time using only a washcloth to scrub the skin and when I do use soap, it is an herbal soap.

Remember, there is beauty and majesty in natural simplicity.

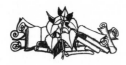

These recipes will make you look ten years younger. (The beeswax and lanolin called for are available at your pharmacy.)

BASIC CLEANSING CREAM: The recipe calls for 2 tablespoons beeswax, 2 ounces lanolin, 2 tablespoons herbal infusion water (instructions follow), 3/8 cup of olive oil and 1/8 ounce of scented oil (if desired). Melt lanolin and beeswax in a double boiler over low heat. When melted, add the olive oil. Remove from heat and stir in scented oil. Stir continuously until cool. It will thicken and become creamy. Store in a screw-top jar.

Use this cream to clean your face. Apply a small amount, massage into face. Place a hot cloth over face. As the cloth cools, rinse it in hot water to heat it up again. Do this several times. Remove all traces of cleanser with a clean tissue. Use herbal infusion to pat on as a skin toner.

BASIC HERBAL INFUSION: Pour 1-1/4 cups boiling water over herb of your choice. Use 3-4 tablespoons fresh herb or 1 teaspoon of dried herb. Use chinaware or earthenware container. Steep 30 minutes and strain. Bottle the mixture in a screw-top container and refrigerate. It keeps about a week. Use cold. This tonic has many beneficial effects, depending on the herb used.

Chamomile: Tones up relaxed muscles.

Fennel: An infusion of the leaves and seeds clears up spots.

Lemon balm: Smooths wrinkles.

Mints: All mints are excellent astringents.

Rosemary: Tightens sagging skin.

Comfrey: Mix with witch hazel as an excellent tonic to
smooth wrinkles.

Thyme: An excellent astringent, it helps to clear acne.

Use the infusion at least twice weekly to get best results. You will notice the effects on the first application.

The next few recipes are good for clearing up skin problems.

LEMON BALM: Lemon balm is good for getting rid of wrinkles. Pour 1 pint of boiling water over a handful of fresh lemon balm and use as a rinse every morning.

TO IMPROVE COMPLEXION: Chicory has long been used as a coffee substitute, but the beautiful blue flowers can be used as a tea to help clear the complexion and give it a healthy glow. Pour 1 cup boiling water over a small handful of chicory flowers. Cover and steep 15 minutes. Strain and sweeten. Drink at least 1 cup a day.

COMPLEXION CARE: To really improve your complexion, place 1 cup calendula leaves and\or flowers into 1 cup olive oil. You can also use any of the vegetable oils in place of the olive oil. Allow the herb to soak for for several days. Strain off the herbs and flowers and smooth the oil gently into the skin at night. This can also be used to heal skin abrasions and cuts. It's good for bruises too.

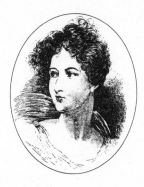

VIOLET LOTION: This lotion has lots of vitamin A, so you know how good it is for the skin. There is no better oil for our skins than almond oil. It smooths, softens, and feeds the skin, and it's great for under the eyes. Place 1/2 cup of fresh violet leaves and 1/2 cup violet flowers in a stainless steel pan. Cover the herbs with almond oil. Place the pan on very, very low heat and leave to steep for about 6 hours, covered. Strain off the flowers/leaves and add 1 ounce of melted beeswax to the almond oil. Stir until mixture is creamy. Test for firmness. If too stiff, add a little more almond oil. Pour into pretty jars and use daily.

ELDER FLOWER BEAUTY BAG: Gather and dry all the elder flowers you can. Make beauty bags of small terry wash cloths folded in a triangle and sewn on machine. Stuff with dried elder flowers and use to wash face and hands to soften and whiten the skin.

SKIN MOISTURIZER: Mix 1 egg yolk and 1 tablespoon glycerin. Smooth on face and let dry. Leave on for 5 minutes before removing.

DRY SKIN LOTION: Put 1 tablespoon castor oil, 1/2 cup mineral oil, 1/2 tablespoon cod-liver oil and 2 tablespoons lecithin in the blender. Now prepare gelatin mix by dissolving 1 tablespoon gelatin in 1/4 cup cold water. Then add 3/4 cup boiling water to the gelatin and let it sit until cool. Add 1/2 cup of this gelatin to the blender mix. Blend until thoroughly mixed. (Keep the gelatin water you have left. You will want to make other lotions with it.) This lotion is good for thick, rough, flaking and chapped skin.

For skin that is wrinkled, add the juice of 1 or 2 leaves of an aloe vera plant and 1 PABA tablet (1000 mg) to the blender mix. (If sensitive to PABA, omit it.) To clear the skin of freckles, add 1/4 cup of lemon juice. If desired, add scented oil to the mix.

HAND LOTION: I use this all over the body. Melt 1 cup solid vegetable shortening, 2 tablespoons anhydrous lanolin, and 1/4 ounce of beeswax. Remove from heat and add 1/2 cup of olive or almond oil and 1/8 ounce of scented oil. Mix well and let cool. When the mixture has cooled and is solid, stir it well. If too stiff, add more oil. If too soft, add more melted beeswax. One way to test the texture is to place one tablespoon of the lotion in the refrigerator. After the mixture has cooled completely, check for thickness. Put in attractive jar and use daily.

Caution: Please test for allergic reactions to the lanolin. If you have allergic reactions to wearing wool, chances are you will have a reaction to the use of lanolin. If you are sensitive to the lanolin, leave that out of the recipe and substitute almond oil for the olive oil. Almond oil is a great moisturizer and can be used in place of the lanolin.

SKIN LOTION: Mix 1/3 cup of rose water, 1/3 cup glycerin, 1/3 cup lemon juice and shake well. Use after your bath. This will help to heal sun-damaged skin. This is a good lotion if you do a lot of outdoor chores.

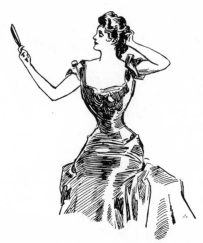

SKIN SOFTENER: Apply almond oil to the skin as a lotion to soften rough skin.

AFTER WINTER PICKUP: Steam the face with peppermint.(Add peppermint leaves to boiling water and make a towel tent over your head to trap the steam.) Then gently massage the face with the following mixture. Mix 1 unbeaten egg white with a few drops of spirit of camphor. Add enough warm milk to make a paste. Put on the face and let dry. Rinse well and blot skin to dry.

SKIN LOTION: Soak 4 tablespoons cracked flax seed for 24 hours in a pint of warm water. Bring to a boil and simmer 15 minutes. Strain off the flax seed and add 3 ounces of glycerin and 1 pint of vinegar. Bring just to boiling point and remove from heat. Several drops of scented oil may be added at this time, if desired. Beat extremely well as the glycerin has a tendency to separate. This is a very good lotion for treating dry skin.

OILY SKIN LOTION: Take 1/2 cup of your gelatin mix liquid (see "Dry Skin Lotion"recipe), 1 tablet of 500 mg vitamin C, 1 multiple vitamin tablet, 1 teaspoon of glycerin, 1 teaspoon of seaweed and place in the blender. Add 1 aspirin if you have bags under the eyes. For sagging skin, add 1/4 teaspoon alum (it helps firm up the skin).

TREATMENT FOR OILY SKIN: Pour 1 cup boiling water over 1 tablespoon of coltsfoot. Allow to steep 30 minutes. Strain and use as a wash for oily skin. Use daily until improvement is noticed.

TREATMENT FOR OILY SKIN: White yarrow is an excellent astringent. So, if you have oily skin try this. Pour 1 cup boiling water over 1 teaspoon of dried yarrow. Let steep for 15 minutes. Strain. Dip a cloth in the hot yarrow water and apply to the face. Let the cloth stay on your face until it is cool. Reapply as needed, depending on how oily your skin is. Apply up to four times for extremely oily skin. It is also a good cleanser, so you can pour it in your bath water if you like.

TO REMOVE FRECKLES: Mix equal parts of lemon juice and buttermilk. Rub on the freckled area. Apply daily and leave on for 30 minutes. Rinse and apply almond or olive oil as a moisturizer. Leave the moisturizer on overnight. Repeat as needed until freckles are gone.

FRECKLE REMOVER: To clear the skin and remove freckles, take 1 handful of elder flowers and leaves and add to 1 pint of boiling water. Let steep 1-1/2 hours. Strain off the leaves/flowers and reheat the liquid. Dip clean cloth in the liquid and use as compress.

SUN SPOTS: To remove sun spots, apply the juice of aloe vera. This could take several months of use before you get results. Aloe vera also removes old scars and helps prevent new scars if it is put on cuts or burns immediately.

SKIN DISCOLORATIONS: Yogurt will bleach the skin. Apply before bed and rinse off the following morning. Yogurt is good for almost everything, so keep plenty on hand to eat and use medicinally.

TO LIGHTEN SKIN DISCOLORATIONS: Separate an egg. Take the egg white and mix it with an equal amount of lemon juice. Beat just until mixed. Place mixture in a custard cup and place in a pan of hot water. Place over low heat. Beat constantly until mixture forms a custard-like consistency. Cool and apply to clean face. Wear overnight.

TO BLEACH YELLOW-TINTED SKIN: Crush a handful of fresh cranberries to extract the juice. Rub into neck and face. Leave on overnight and rinse off in the morning.

SALLOW SKIN: Mix 1 teaspoon soya powder and 1 tablespoon of plain yogurt. Apply to face and allow to stay on for about 30 minutes. Rinse well. If dryness occurs, pat on a thin layer of olive or almond oil.

DULL SKIN COLOR: This recipe dissolves the top layer of dry skin. Saturate clean cloth with pineapple juice and place on the skin as a compress. Leave on at least 30 minutes. Rinse face gently. Break open a vitamin E capsule and apply to the face. Leave on overnight.

    Caution: This recipe is not for everybody. My daughter is extremely allergic to pineapple and can not even touch the juice. Please try a skin patch test before applying to the face. It works well for those that can use it, but again try the test before use.

CLOGGED PORES: Put a large handful of chopped parsley into an earthenware bowl. Pour 1 cup boiling water over the parsley. Cover, and let steep until it reaches room temperature. Strain and apply the liquid to the face as a compress for about 15 minutes. Use daily. This really clears up the complexion.

ACNE TREATMENT: Dilute some liquid hand soap and apply a thin layer to the face. Leave on overnight and it will help to dry up eruptions. *Caution:* This can dry the skin out pretty fast, so I wouldn't use it over once a week. Extra-dry skin can aggravate acne and you do not want to add to the problem.

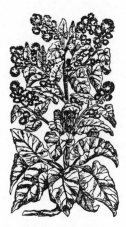

Burdock (Artium lappa)

ACNE TREATMENT: Burdock is a great astringent, great for removing excess oil from the skin. Use it faithfully every day if your skin is oily. It may take several weeks before you notice an improvement. Put 2 handfuls of burdock roots and leaves in 2 cups of water. Bring to a quick boil using a stainless steel or glass pot. Lower heat and simmer 10 minutes. Dip clean cloth into liquid and use as a compress until the cloth cools. Repeat this, keeping the liquid hot, for about 15 minutes.

ACNE TREATMENT: Make a paste of baking soda and water. Apply to the face and leave on for 5 minutes. Rinse off with apple cider vinegar. Rinse again with clear water. Apply a coating of vitamin E oil to your face and leave on overnight.

TREATMENT OF ACNE: Clean face thoroughly. Apply fresh onion juice to the area. Leave on for 15 minutes. Rinse well. Use daily.

TREATMENT OF ACNE: Because thyme is such a good astringent, it can be used to help clear up acne. Pour 1-1/2 cups of boiling water over 3-4 tablespoons of dried thyme. Let steep 30 minutes. Strain and bottle the liquid. Keep refrigerated. Teenagers with acne problems could use this daily as a facial rinse.

BLEMISHES: Rub the face with a crushed strawberry. Leave it on for about 15 minutes. Rinse thoroughly with warm, then cold water. This will help to clear blemishes. *Caution:* Many people are allergic to strawberries. Try a patch test before proceeding to use the facial treatment.

PEPPERMINT CARE: Peppermint tea applied to the face is a good astringent. Soak a clean cloth and apply to the face as a compress.

FACIAL SCRUB: To fight blackheads, moisten a handful of finely ground cornmeal and rub into face for about 5 minutes. Rinse the face and apply a moisturizer.

FACIAL CLEANER: Cook carrots in as little water as possible. When tender, mash thoroughly and apply to the face as a mask. Leave on for 15 minutes and rinse. This is good for treating acne as well. This treatment adds vitamin A to the skin and that helps to prevent wrinkles.

BEAUTY PACK: Apply a paste made of sea salt and water. Keep on face for 20 minutes, then rinse thoroughly.

FENNEL AND COLTSFOOT FACIAL PACK: This soothes, softens, closes pores, and tones the skin. It also helps to minimize wrinkles and to fight acne. Pour 1/2 cup of boiling water over 2 tablespoons of dried coltsfoot leaves and 1 tablespoon dried fennel leaves. Cover and steep for 10 minutes. Strain well, keeping the liquid. Add the liquid to 1/2 cup of yogurt and a handful of oatmeal to make a paste. Wash face thoroughly and cover face with a hot cloth for a few minutes. Cover eyes with damp cotton pads and spread warmed paste over the face. Leave on for 10 minutes. Wash off with warm water that has a little lemon juice added to it.

BEAUTY MASK: Puree 1 red or green sweet pepper in your blender. Apply the mixture to your face. Leave the mask on for 15 minutes. Rinse off with cool water and apply vitamin E oil as an overnight help. The sweet pepper works as a good cleanser.

BRACING SKIN CLEANSER (CAN BE USED BY MEN AND WOMEN): Squeeze 1 orange and 3 lemons. Add 1 cup of rose water, the juice of 1 cucumber and 1 cup of vodka. Apply to the face as a rinse. Men use this as a bracing after-shave splash.

TO CONDITION THE SKIN: Pound 1/2 cup each pumpkin seeds, gourd seeds, and cucumber seeds until reduced to a powder. Add enough cream to make a thin paste. Add a few drops of oil of lemon. Massage into skin and leave on overnight if possible. Wash off with warm water.

SKIN TIGHTENER: Mix together 2 tablespoons of unbeaten egg whites, 1 tablespoon powdered milk and 1/2 teaspoon of honey. Beat until well-blended. Apply to face and allow to dry. Rinse with warm water and blot dry. Rinse face with herbal astringent.

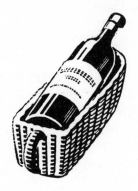

LIP CARE: Bring 2 cups of white wine to boiling. Add a small piece of gum benzoin. Slow boil for 30 minutes. Put 15 drops of this in a glass of water. It will turn milky and have a very good smell. Apply the liquid to the lips. The preparation will bring the blood to the surface and make your lips a natural red. This can also be used as a splash for the face. Splash on and allow it to dry. It gives color and a nice clear complexion. It's also good for freckles, pimples and skin eruptions.

LIP BALM: To make your own lip balm for chapped lips, simply melt 1-1/2 ounces of beeswax over hot water (you could use a double boiler). Stir in 1 ounce of honey. Beat in 2 ounces of olive oil. Continue stirring until cool. Put in a wide mouth jar. Apply as needed to prevent chapped lips.

TASTY LIP BALM: This is great to use to protect your lips during cold weather. Young girls like to wear it all the time. Put it in small tins to carry in your purse.

Mix together 1/2 cup almond oil, 1/4 cup cocoa butter, and 1/4 cup of coconut oil. Melt all the ingredients over a low fire. Stir in 1 tablespoon of honey and 2 ounces of beeswax. After the beeswax is melted, add 1-1/2 teaspoons of any natural flavoring. Vanilla, cherry, lemon, orange, coconut or any of the flavorings you have in your spice cabinet will do fine. Mix completely and test for firmness. It needs to be firm, so you may have to add more melted beeswax to get the desired consistency.

SAGE AND VIOLET CREAM: Use this to alleviate cold sores. It also soothes and protects chapped lips.

Put 2 tablespoons each of fresh violet leaves and fresh sage in 4 tablespoons of almond oil into a jar that can be closed tightly. Close and place in a warm, sunny area for 1 month. Shake daily. After 1 month, strain the liquid into an earthenware or glass bowl and add 4 more tablespoons of almond oil. Melt 4 tablespoons of beeswax and add to the almond oil mixture, stirring until mixture is cool and has consistency. Store tightly closed, in a cool place. Apply as needed to treat cold sores or protect lips.

LIP GLOSS: Melt 1 tablespoon beeswax over hot water. Add 5 tablespoons olive oil. Add 1/4 teaspoon alkanet root. It makes a deep burgundy gloss. Strain and put in glass jar. You can leave out the alkanet root and add leftover commercial lipstick. Create your own colors by mixing several different shades of lipstick into the gloss.

REFRESHING MOUTH WASH: Mix 1 teaspoon each of peppermint, rosemary and lavender. Use 1 teaspoon of the mixture to 1 cup of boiling water. Steep 15 minutes. Strain and use as a mouth wash.

MOUTH WASH: Mix 2 teaspoons sugar, 3 drops peppermint oil, 3/4 teaspoon of boric acid solution and 4 cups of water. Add food coloring if desired. Put into a quart bottle. Shake to mix well. Use as a mouth wash and breath freshener. *Caution:* Do not drink.

ANGELICA MOUTH WASH: This freshens the mouth and sweetens the breath. Use twice daily for most effective action. Pour 2 cups boiling water over 3 tablespoons of angelica seeds. Add peppermint, lemon verbena, caraway or rosemary for extra strength. Adding a little orris root will perfume the breath with the scent of violets. Cover and steep until cool. Strain and store in tightly closed container. Use as a gargle to rinse the mouth.

SPICY MOUTH WASH: Add 3 drops of cinnamon oil, 2 drops of clove oil, 2 teaspoons sugar and 3/4 teaspoon of boric acid solution to 4 cups of water. Put in quart container and shake well. Add coloring if desired.

BREATH FRESHENER: Add 1 tablespoon allspice to a cup of hot water and use as a gargle.

EYE MAKEUP REMOVER: If you really feel it necessary to wear eye makeup, remove every day to avoid infection of the eyes. Use safflower oil for a non-allergenic aid.

NAIL CARE: To soften cuticles and strengthen the nails, mix together 3 tablespoons of almond oil, 3 tablespoons raw linseed oil, and 3 tablespoons of honey. Massage into nails and cuticles.

HORSETAIL NAIL STRENGTHENER: This is a wonderful herbal way to strengthen brittle or splitting nails. Pour 2-1/2 cups of water over 6 tablespoons of dried horsetail stems, using a stainless steel pan. Allow to infuse for about 4 hours. Place on heat and bring to a boil. Reduce heat to simmer. Simmer, covered, gently for 30 minutes. Remove from heat and allow to steep another 30 minutes before straining off the horsetail stems. Every two days, soak fingernails in warm sunflower oil for 15 minutes, then in the horsetail mixture for another 15 minutes. Store the infusion in a tightly closed container. It really strengthens the nails.

SPLITTING NAILS: Eating plenty of cucumber or drinking the juice of cucumbers seems to help correct this problem.

STIMULATING AFTER-SHAVE: Mix 1 cup each of peppermint, yarrow flowers, fresh or dried lavender flowers, and 3 cups of sage leaves. Place in a large jar and cover with rubbing alcohol. Let steep for 2 weeks. Strain and add 1 cup of water. If the skin is dry, add 2 tablespoons of glycerin or almond oil. This also makes a wonderful massage for aching muscles.

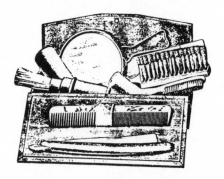

AFTER-SHAVE LOTION: Add 1 ounce dried lavender flowers and 1 ounce of sage to 2 cups of witch hazel. Place in a tightly closed jar and let sit for 1 week in a very warm area. Strain and rebottle. Very invigorating and has a nice clean scent.

STYPTIC LOTION: Mix 1/4 cup of water, 1/2 teaspoon of alum and 1/8 teaspoon glycerin. Shake well each time you use the lotion. Apply to nicks after shaving to stop bleeding.

CREAM DEODORANT: Melt in a pan together 3 tablespoons each of baking soda, petroleum jelly, and orris root powder (or corn starch). Add a few drops of scented oil. Apply for underarm protection.

DEODORANT: Put 1 tablespoon of powdered alum, 1 tablespoon rubbing alcohol and 1/8 ounce scented oil in 1-3/4 cups of water. Place in a spray bottle for use.

SCENTED BATH LOTION: Use rubbing alcohol or witch hazel. Add 1/2 cup each of mint, lemon balm, rosemary and lavender to 1 quart of alcohol or witch hazel. (Mix the herbs of your choice to make this bath lotion.) Let steep in the sun for 2 weeks, shaking every day. It will turn a nice herby green. Strain, place in a tightly closed container and label. Use as a fragrant rub after bathing.

BATH SALTS: Mix together 1/2 cup of salt, 1/2 cup Epsom salts, and 1/2 cup baking soda. Mix well, adding food coloring and scented oil if desired. Keep tightly closed. Add to bath water by tablespoons to desired strength. It makes a very soothing and relaxing bath, as well as being good for your skin.

SCENTED BATH POWDER: Mix 1 ounce of orris root, 1/2 table-spoon powdered cloves, and 1 ounce of powdered sage. Add 2 ounces of corn starch and mix well. To make different scents, simply add the herb of your choice. Use powdered herbs if possible, otherwise grind as fine as you can. Keep tightly closed to retain scent.

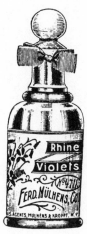

BATH POWDERS: Simply add a few drops of scented oil to corn starch or arrowroot. Apply after bath. Add the same scent that you use to make your perfume.

) MAKE YOUR OWN PERFUME: Use 1/2 cup of essen-
ny scent or mix), 1/2 cup powdered orris root, 3 cups
vodka and mix well. Pour in pretty bottles and store in cool, dark
place. It is really fun to try mixing scents for gifts. You can also mix
a special one for yourself, one that everyone will come to associate
only with you.

PREPARE YOUR OWN ESSENTIAL OILS: Place 3 tablespoons
of your favorite chosen herbs, crushed, into a pint of vegetable oil
in a quart container. Add 1 tablespoon of plain vinegar, not malt
vinegar. Cap jar and try to place in the sun. If done during the winter, place in a very warm spot. Let steep 1 week, then strain and
add additional dried herbs. Repeat for 2 more weeks. Strain and
bottle. Store in a dark place.

FOOT BATH: Pour 1 quart of boiling water over 4-5 handfuls of
silver birch bark and steep for 30 minutes. Strain off the bark and
pour into the foot bath. This can also be used in your bath water as
it helps to soothe aching muscles and helps the pain of arthritis.

FOOT BATH: Soak your tired and aching feet! It really does feel
good if you throw in a handful of your favorite herb. Lavender,
calendula leaves, and all the mints are very refreshing.

LAVENDER BATH MIXTURE: Crush and mix 1 ounce of dried
lavender flowers, 1 ounce of dried basil, 2 teaspoons of cinnamon.
Add to 1 pint of witch hazel. Steep for 2 weeks and strain. Add 1/4
cup to bath water or use as an after-bath splash.

APPLE BATH ADDITION: Pour 1-1/2 pints of boiling water over
1/4 cup of dried apple slices, 1/2 teaspoon of cinnamon, and 1/2
teaspoon of whole cloves. Steep for 30 minutes. Use in bath water
for a very refreshing bath.

HERBAL LOVE BATH: This is to pamper yourself when you're
down. Mix 7 cups of lavender, 6 cups of rosemary, 5 cups rose
petals, 4 cups of lovage, 3 cups verbena leaves, 1 cup each of
thyme, mint, marjoram, and orris powder. Put in a container and
keep tightly closed. To use, put 1/4 cup of the mixture in a muslin

bag and tie securely. Boil the bath ball in 1 quart of water for 10 minutes. Add to bath water and scrub with the bath ball. Makes a really nice gift.

SCENTED BATH FOR MEN: Mix equal parts of lavender and pine needles. Boil and steep for 15 minutes. Strain and add to bath water. Lavender, verbena, nutmeg, geranium, lemon balm, and thyme are all good to add for a manly scent. If desired, you may add 1 tablespoon (or more) of the herb mixture to enhance the scent.

APHRODISIAC: This is a good tea to drink after you've thoroughly relaxed with your love bath. Make it out of any of the following herbs: orange blossoms, rose petals, chamomile, bee balm, fennel, licorice, ginseng, or any of the mints. To use, put 1 teaspoon of any of the herbs (or a mixture of these herbs) in 1 cup of boiling water. Let steep 15 minutes. Strain and sweeten with honey. Ginger and lemon may be added to the tea to your taste.

QUICK AND EASY POTPOURRI FOR YOUR BATHROOM: Mix dried rose buds and petals with basil, thyme, lavender, and other herbs of your choice. Add spices such as ground cinnamon, cloves, allspice, dried lemon or orange peel, ground orris root and a few drops of scented oil. Age in a tightly closed jar 4-8 weeks. This also makes a nice gift.

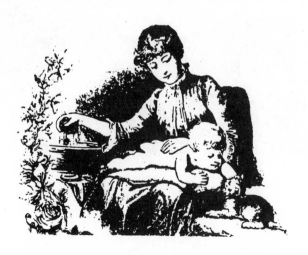

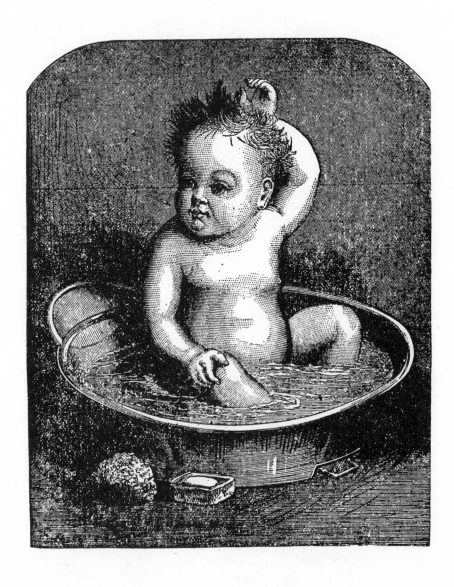

·3·

Hair Care

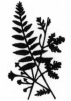

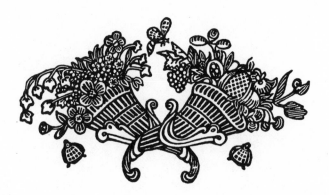

Hair styles come and go. The hair has to be healthy to withstand the stress we put it through daily. Diet plays an important part in keeping our Crowning Glory healthy. Simplify your diet and your hair benefits. Use some of these recipes as a start on getting healthier hair.

HERBAL SHAMPOOS: Put 2 tablespoons dried soapwort, 1 tablespoon chamomile flowers, and 2 teaspoons borax in a large jar or container made out of pottery or chinaware. Pour 2-1/2 cups of boiling water over the herb mixture and cover tightly. Let steep for several days. Shake the container every once in a while. Strain, discarding the herbs. This will not be as soapy as commercial shampoo, but it's cleansing qualities are undeniable. Add a few sprigs of lavender or lime blossoms before covering to give a natural delicate fragrance. Soapwort is nothing more then wild sweet william, so it is easy to grab a few handfuls to make the shampoo.

YUCCA-ROOT SHAMPOO (ALSO CALLED SOAPWEED): Dig or purchase the yucca roots. Chop into small pieces and pulverize into a pulp (using a hammer or blender). When the substance has changed from white to pale amber, it is ready to use. You can dry for later use by spreading the material on a clean surface in the sun until all moisture has evaporated. The pulp should no longer feel sticky.

When using this shampoo, make sure that your hands are free from grease, or the shampoo won't lather. Place a small amount of

the root in a cheesecloth bag. Wet and lather to wa
the hair shiny and silky.

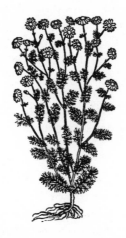

Wild Chamomile (Matricaria chamomilla)

CHAMOMILE SHAMPOO: Make herbal infusion by pouring 4 cups boiling water over 5 tablespoons of chamomile flowers. Cover and steep 30 minutes. Strain and add 4 ounces castile soap flakes. Makes 1 quart of shampoo. This is the favorite shampoo around our house. You can purchase the castile soap flakes from any of the companies that sell herbs. It's easy to make and easy on the hair.

SHAMPOO SUBSTITUTE: Beat an egg and massage into scalp twice each week. Rinse with vinegar water, then rinse with plain water. This is a good treatment for your hair. Leaves it shiny and healthy.

SHAMPOO FOR COARSE HAIR: Put 1 ounce of white oak bark into 1 cup of water. Bring to a boil and reduce heat to simmer. Simmer for 20 minutes. Strain and add to 1 ounce of liquid castile soap. Now add 3 tablespoons of the herb soap to 1 teaspoon of honey and 1 beaten egg. Shampoo hair. Rinse well with apple cider vinegar rinse. This one is great for older people to use. My mother used this and her hair was beautiful. It seems to take the coarseness out of graying or silver hair.

NETTLE ROSEMARY SHAMPOO: This is a very fragrant stimulant for the scalp. It prevents dandruff and promotes hair growth. In a small stainless steel pan, place 2 handfuls of soapwort. Pour 1-1/2 cups of water over the soapwort. Bring to a boil, lower heat, and simmer for 10 minutes. Remove from the heat and cover. Allow to steep until cool. Strain into a bottle that closes tightly. Place a handful of young chopped nettle leaves and 1-1/2 table-spoons of chopped fresh rosemary in in a bowl. Pour 1 cup boiling water over the chopped herbs. Allow to infuse 30 minutes. Cool and strain into the soapwort mixture. Shake the shampoo before using.

IF YOU MUST USE COMMERCIAL SHAMPOO, THEN FOL-LOW THIS RECIPE: Use a ratio of 2 tablespoons of apple cider vinegar to 2 cups of water to make a final rinse for hair after shampoo. This counteracts the alkaline affect of commercial shampoo.

HAIR RINSE: Pour 4 cups of boiling water over 2 tablespoons of the chosen herb. Cover and let stand 30 minutes. Strain and use as a hair rinse. It is a simple matter to make a hair rinse from of any of the following:
  Sage: A good conditioner.
  Fennel: Also conditions.
  Parsley: Clears up dandruff.
  Chamomile: Lightens hair, promotes growth.
  Rosemary: Darkens hair, leaves a delicious fragrance.
  Nettle leaves (Use dried): Excellent to treat dandruff.

HAIR SETTING LOTION (THIS IS GOOD FOR LIGHT HAIR): This lotion adds body as well as setting the hair. Add 1 teaspoon of powdered milk to 1/2 cup of warm water. Apply to hair and set. To achieve a stiffer set, add more powdered milk. This works just as well if you add orris root powder instead of using powdered milk.

SETTING GEL: Aloe vera makes a very good hair setting gel. It dries quickly and leaves the hair shiny. This works well with curly hair. It adds a shine as well as working as a setting gel.

HAIR TONICS: Massage diluted lemon juice into the scalp at least once a week before shampooing. This lightens hair and conditions the scalp. It's also good to use if you suffer from dandruff.

HAIR TONIC: Mix 2 tablespoons of lemon juice with 1/2 cup of witch hazel. Massage in the scalp after a shampoo.

MINT TONIC: Before you shampoo your hair, massage in the following herbal tea. Put 3 tablespoons of dried mint into 1 cup of water and 1/2 cup of vinegar. Simmer for 15 minutes. Steep until cool. Strain and massage the tea into scalp. Stimulates the scalp.

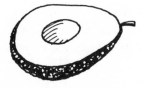

Avocado (Persa americana)

CONDITIONER: Instead of using commercial creme rinses that can do harm, try using this avocado conditioner. Chop an avocado in the blender until very fine. Massage into the hair for 5 minutes. Rinse thoroughly. Leaves the hair shiny and bright.

OILY HAIR: Use this as a final rinse for oily hair. Put 1/2 cup of rosemary into 1-1/2 cups of water. Bring to a full boil, then simmer for 15 minutes. Let sit 24 hours, covered. Strain, bottle and use daily for 1 week. Thereafter, use at least once weekly.

DANDRUFF TREATMENT: In a separate container, mix 1 cup burdock, 1 cup peach tree leaves, 1 cup chamomile, 1/2 cup sage leaves. Pour 2 quarts of cider vinegar into a gallon jar. Add the herb mixture to the cider vinegar. Let stand for 2 weeks. Strain and apply morning and evening. Do not rinse off. Let dry on hair. Wait until the next day to rinse it out. There is no need to use any soap or shampoo to rinse out the treatment. Using plain water will wash this treatment along with the dirt from your hair. This works quickly on dandruff. To darken the hair with this recipe, add 1 cup of hop flowers to the herbs before allowing them to steep in the vinegar.

CONTROL DANDRUFF: This is a great rinse and helps to control dandruff too. Pour 1 pint of boiling water over 1/2 cup of chopped parsley. Let stand 30 minutes. Massage into scalp and allow to stay on 15 minutes. Use as final rinse.

DANDRUFF TREATMENT: Add 4 tablespoons of dried nettle to 1 pint boiling water. Steep overnight. Strain and add 1 cup of apple cider vinegar. Massage into the scalp. Can also be used as a face rinse to get rid of oily skin. Apple cider vinegar is great to use for scalp treatments, facial treatments or simply to add to your bath. It helps to keep the skin clear if you drink a little vinegar water a couple times a week. Add honey and you keep your whole body toned up.

DANDRUFF TREATMENT: Dissolve 10 aspirins (5 grains each) in 1 cup warm water. Massage into scalp for about 10 minutes. Rinse thoroughly. Add a vinegar rinse as an extra help after rinsing aspirin out completely. Use after every shampoo if necessary for awhile.

DARKENS HAIR: Pour 1 cup of boiling water over 3 tablespoons of rosemary. Let stand overnight. Strain and use as a final rinse. This also enhances curly hair. As a bonus, it really makes the hair glossy and leaves a nice smell.

DARKENS GRAY HAIR: To darken gray hair, pour 1 cup boiling water over 4 tablespoons of dried sage. Let steep overnight. Combine with 1 cup commercial tea and work into hair every night until desired color is reached. A male friend swears by this treatment. We teased him for years about his premature gray hair until he started using this treatment. Native Americans have used sage tea as a treatment for gray hair for centuries.

LIGHTEN HAIR: To lighten hair, mix several tablespoons of lemon juice to 1 cup of water. Apply as final rinse. Let hair dry in the sun if possible. This is great for natural blondes and it will add highlights to darker hair.

HAIR RINSE FOR REDHEADS: There is no better rinse for redheads than pot marigold (*calendula*). Have a basin ready to catch the rinse as you pour it over your hair, because you will need to repeat the rinse. To prepare the rinse, pour 2 cups boiling water over 1/2 cup of calendula flowers. Let stand 30 minutes. Strain off the flowers and use the liquid as a final rinse after shampooing. Repeat rinse at least 20 times. Let dry in the sun. It really makes the hair gleam.

HAIR COLORING FOR BRUNETTES: Mix together 1/4 cup of powdered chamomile and 1/2 cup of powdered henna. Add just enough boiling water to make a paste along with 1 tablespoon of vinegar. Allow the paste to cool. Put on rubber gloves before massaging into clean wet hair. Be sure to comb the paste through the hair and apply it evenly. Pile up the hair and cover it with a plastic bag. Wrap a thick towel over the plastic to hold in the heat. Leave on at least 30 minutes. Remove towel and rinse hair until the water runs clear. Allow to dry in sunshine. Any stains on face or hands can be removed with lemon juice. This mixture has a tendency to add red overtones to the hair, so you might want to pretest it. Do not use if you have white, blond, or gray hair as it will turn those colors a brassy orange. It does add nice highlights to dark brunettes.

BLOND HAIR: To prepare the rinse, pour 1 quart of boiling water over 1/2 cup of chamomile flowers. Let steep 30 minutes. Add the juice of 2 lemons to really lighten hair and add highlights. Have a basin ready to catch the rinse as you will need to repeat the rinsing. Pour directly onto clean hair as a rinse. Continue pouring over hair at least 20 times.

TO SPEED HAIR GROWTH: Boil 1/2 cup of peach seeds (these are found inside of the pit) in 2 cups of vinegar until thick. Strain and massage into scalp. Rinse well. This seems to stimulate the scalp. Many times changing your diet will promote hair growth, if it is not an hereditary condition. Also, if medication is being taken, people have a tendency to lose hair at an alarming rate. Get your diet back to normal as fast as possible after an illness and try to ingest as few chemicals as possible. A simple, natural diet does more to get your body back into good condition than any other action.

THINNING HAIR: Dietary supplements can help with thinning hair. It helps to take a multi-vitamin and mineral supplement that contains 25 mg of each of the major B vitamins. Along with the vitamin capsule you should be taking about 1/2 cup of brewers yeast in any form you can get. Add it to the liquids you drink and sprinkle on the foods that you eat but make sure you have at least 1/2 cup per day. This is especially true if you are recovering from an illness.

If loss of hair is a natural condition for you due to hereditary conditions (as it is for many men), then I would advise you to keep your diet healthy, so as to have the best looking scalp in the neighborhood. If you are a woman whose hair is starting to thin due to loss of estrogen production, there are herbs you can take to simulate estrogen in your system and to stimulate the adrenal glands. Mix equal parts of wild yam root, licorice, mother wort, black cohosh, chamomile, valerian root and skullcap. Take 2 daily. I have taken this mixture for years, ever since I had a hysterectomy at the age of 28. After taking prescription estrogen for several years and putting up with the side-effects, I knew I could do better. And I did.

TREATMENT FOR BALDNESS: Mix together 1 teaspoon oil of rosemary, 5 drops oil of lemongrass, 4 ounces of olive oil. Rub small amount into scalp every night for a week. Do not shampoo until the end of the week.

SHAMPOO TREATMENT FOR BALDNESS: This shampoo will stimulate the scalp and promote hair growth. Pour 1 cup boiling water over 1/2 ounce of dried rosemary. Let steep 24 hours. Strain and add 1/2 cup castile shampoo. Shake well before using. Should be used every other night and allowed to stay on the scalp for 15 minutes before rinsing off. If your hair is thinning, stay away from commercial shampoos. This has been used with success by a friend and seemed to help a lot. It could have been the fact that no commercial shampoo was used along with the stimulation from the rosemary.

THIS IS SAID TO REALLY PROMOTE HAIR GROWTH: Mix 2 teaspoons of cayenne pepper with 1 cup of olive oil. Massage into the area that is thinning on a daily basis. Continue treatment. You will get results in a few days. I know of several men who have been using this treatment and it does seem to help. But when the treatment stops, so does the hair growth. Keep up the treatment if you do obtain good results with use.

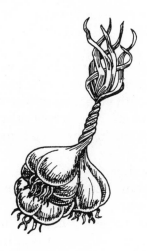

Garlic (Allium sativum)

GARLIC TREATMENT FOR BALD SPOTS: Rub a halved clove of garlic over bald or thinning areas of the scalp. Repeat at least three times daily. Allow the area to dry before rinsing off. You should notice results in a few weeks.

THINNING HAIR: Rub the scalp with a freshly cut onion until the scalp is red. Massage in a small amount of vitamin E oil or honey and rinse off with rosemary tea. Towel dry the hair. This should be done every morning and evening.

THINNING HAIR: Mix 1/4 cup of cayenne pepper with 1 cup of vodka. Steep for about 2 weeks. Strain and rub into the scalp morning and night. *Caution:* Do not get near the eyes. This seems to help as much as the olive oil and cayenne mixture. Again, the hair growth slows down and stops if treatment is stopped. It is not as greasy as the olive oil treatment and seems to suit some people better than the olive oil.

TREATMENT FOR THINNING HAIR: Place 1 large, sliced onion in 1 pint of brandy. Steep for 2 weeks. Strain and add 1 cup of water. Rub in the scalp twice daily.

BALD PATCHES: Rub the bald areas with apple cider vinegar using a soft toothbrush 2 times daily. It will stimulate new hair growth.

Vinegar is a good treatment for almost any scalp condition. You should use it as a final rinse regardless of hair type. Keep a shampoo bottle filled with vinegar and water mixture in the shower to have handy at all times. It can be a pain to have to mix a rinse every time you need it. Just use as a final rinse after shampooing.

I remember growing up and using homemade soap as a shampoo. There is nothing better really than that homemade soap. It leaves the hair shiny and squeaky clean. The recipe that I call a miracle soap is in the following chapter and contains olive oil, coconut oil and shortening, so you can see that it would be a wonderful treatment for normal or dry hair. My daughter, who has oily hair, also uses it and it seems to help with an oily condition. And I might add that my husband loves it as a shampoo.

What could be easier than using the same soap to wash and shampoo with? It seems to give the hair body, leaves it shiny and healthy looking, and you can add any scent you want.

•4•

Skin Care

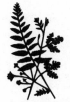

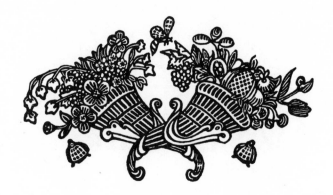

Taking care of our skin is very important. The skin, intact, is our first defense against any invasion of foreign matter that can be harmful to our system. The skin is considered a third kidney because we excrete toxins through the pores just as we do through the kidneys. We also ingest many chemicals and toxins through the skin, so it is important that we pay attention to what we use to clean, soothe, or heal our skin. The skin also plays an important part in regulating our body temperature.

Most injuries to our skin are simple and taking care of them is easy. Cleaning any wound or puncture immediately following an injury should be the first step. Seek medical help if necessary. Keeping the area clean during healing prevents many problems from developing later on.

Some of the skin problems are indicative of internal problems, such as an improper diet. Diet plays an important part in caring for our skin. If we stick to a simple, natural diet and use only natural products to clean or protect us, we will have a much healthier immune system, one that is better able to deal with the viruses or bacteria that we come into contact with daily. Keeping the immune system healthy should be the major goal in seeking a healthy lifestyle.

One of the first ways you can begin to live a healthy lifestyle is to make your own soap. Many people would like to, but think that it is a difficult thing to do. The whole procedure takes about 1-

1/2 hours from start to finish. I make it as I need it and only have to do so a couple of times yearly.

There are no artificial chemicals in this homemade soap and that really is the first step in being chemical-free. The ingredients are simple and there are only a few tools involved. You will need a wooden spoon; a wide-mouth, glass 1/2 gallon jar; several flat containers that you can line with plastic wrap (you could use several shoe boxes if desired); an enamel or iron pot in which to "cook" the soap, and a photography or dairy thermometer. The temperature is important when making soap, so get a good thermometer that registers as low as 95-98 degrees.

There are several rules to follow when making your soap:

1. Get your containers ready by either greasing them or lining them with plastic wrap. Do this first so that they are ready when needed.

2. Never use aluminum to prepare your soap. Always use enamel, stainless steel, or iron containers. You use the wide-mouth glass container to mix your lye solution in, but you will need a container of enamel or iron to "cook" your soap.

3. Never allow your curing soap to sit in a drafty area as this will make your finished product hard and flinty. I cover mine with several thicknesses of newspaper and then cover with a folded blanket for several days.

4. Make sure your molds are at least 1-1/2 to 2 inches thick. If the mold is too thin, it will cause the soap to curl. If it is too thick, it will make the soap too big and it will be difficult to hold. To add scent to your soap, add the scented oil right before you pour the soap into your molds. Any of the scented oils will do. I like to use the vanilla scent for my own personal use, but any that you prefer will do great. Try using a fruity or flower scent. Sometimes kids like the smell of peppermint and this works great too.

You will need to add about 2 tablespoons of the scented oil to each batch. Add more if stronger scent is desired. The scented oils that you add can be of help in treating skin disorders. Lavender oil is an excellent astringent. Adding olive or almond oil is great for dry skin. Thyme oil acts as a deodorant aid. If you prefer, you don't need to add any oils. The plain soap alone is great for your skin because it has no artificial additives in it.

5. *When adding the lye to the cold water, please do so slowly and carefully.* I never would make it when the kids were around because I was afraid that they would get into the solution when my back was turned. I have since learned that kittens are very curious and you need to watch your pets if you make it outdoors. I had a very close call with one of my kittens, so please take certain precautions. *Wear rubber gloves and do not breathe in the fumes.* The mixture will heat up when you are pouring the lye in the water so be sure to use very cold water. *Stir very slowly to avoid splattering and burning yourself.* The splatters will also cause damage to counter tops so you may want to do this procedure outdoors. Making the soap outdoors will also cut down on the fumes.

If you happen to splash any of the solution on your skin, rinse off immediately and rinse the area with vinegar. Vinegar will neutralize the lye somewhat. Continue stirring until the lye crystals are completely dissolved. You will need to place the jar in a pan (or sink) filled with cold water to bring the temperature of the lye solution back down to 90-95 degrees. After that temperature is reached, slowly add the lye solution to the oil.

BASIC SOAP: This recipe is for the basic soap. To make your lye solution, add 13 ounces of lye to 5 cups of cold water in your wide-mouth jar, stirring until your lye crystals are completely dissolved. Place jar in cold water to start bringing the temperature down to about 90-95 degrees. In an enamel pan, slowly melt 6 pounds of lard. Place that enamel container in cold water and bring that temperature down to about 120-130 degrees. When temperatures for both solutions are right, slowly add the lye solution to the melted lard, stirring constantly with a wooden spoon. Keep stirring continuously for about 30 minutes. Add the scented oil and pour into greased molds. Cool overnight.

If you use just one container for a mold instead of individual molds, you need to cut the soap into bars the next morning. Remove the soap from the mold after several days. Age the soap for about two weeks before using. Remember that aging only improves your soap.

MIRACLE SOAP: This recipe is great for dry skin. It lathers up wonderfully. I call it my miracle soap because I use it to wash my hair with too and it is great for the skin. This soap does not get hard fast, so don't feel that you have failed if it does not harden quickly. The temperature is important for this recipe and so are the measurements and weights. You might fail if either is incorrect. Make sure you have an accurate scale to weigh your ingredients. If you don't have one, you need to add one to your equipment list. This recipe makes about 7 pounds of soap.

Ingredients needed are:
10-3/4 ounces of lye crystals
4 cups cold water
27 ounces of coconut oil
34 ounces of olive oil
24 ounces of vegetable shortening (NOT lard or butter or margarine)
1/2 ounce scented oil
1 wide-mouth jar
1 enamel or stainless steel pan
1 wooden spoon

Measure 10-3/4 ounces of lye in a plastic container. Slowly and cautiously add the lye to 4 cups of cold water in the wide-mouth jar. (See rule number five on previous page.) Stir until lye crystals are completely dissolved. Place the jar in a shallow pan of cold water to start bringing the temperature of the lye water down to between 95-98 degrees. The temperature cannot be hotter or colder than this for this recipe. Use the thermometer to continue taking the temperature until proper temperature is reached.

This cooling process takes a little time, so place your shortening in the enamel pan and melt that. Add the olive oil and the coconut oil after you have melted the shortening. You may need to place this in cold water to bring the temperature to between 95-98 degrees. If either solution is too hot or too cold, you may have to heat it up or cool it down to proper temperatures. When both solutions are ready, slowly add the lye solution to the oils in a steady stream, stirring constantly.

Keep stirring until the mixture traces. This means that the spoon lifted from the soap mixture will be able to trace a design on the creamy soap. This design will stay visible for several seconds before disappearing. If you have stirred for about 30 minutes and the soap does not trace well, it is still able to be used. It will just take a little more time to harden after you pour it into the molds.

Before pouring into the molds, add the scented oils. Cover your molds with a folded blanket and place them on a level surface, sheltered from any drafts. Allow to set for 24 hours. Uncover and allow to set another 24 hours. If your scale and thermometer read correctly, you should have a batch of beautiful soap. Carefully following instructions and having equipment that reads correctly always ensures a good batch.

This recipe makes soap that is pliable when removed from the molds. At that time, you would be able to make it into different shapes, designs and sizes. It will have the consistency of soft cheese and be easy to roll into balls or shape into animals for the kids. You can become quite artistic in design. A friend of mine even makes hers into suggestive shapes for her husband's personal use. The soap may be easier to carve into shapes after it has had a chance to set more firmly.

In addition to carving, there are many ways to make your soaps more attractive. You can make "soap on a rope" by forming the soap around a knotted cord. To make the soap prettier, select a glass with an attractive design on the bottom and press the bottom of the glass into the soap.

Wrap the seasoned soap in pretty tissue paper, tie with a bright cord or ribbon, and then store it or give it as gifts. I like to line a small box with tissue paper and place three to a box. It's handy to have around if you need to unexpectedly give a gift.

If you plan on using your own herbs to make the soap, you would need to make a strong tea from the herb desired and cool it completely after straining. You can make it the night before and store in the refrigerator overnight. It will not make as strong a scent as the scented oils will. And the scent does disappear completely while you are using the soap.

For a coarser texture, try adding cornmeal or oatmeal that has been ground in the food processor, or grains of pumice to the mixture. This is good for people working on cars, or others who need a grainy soap to remove oils from their hands. Try adding powdered herbs or spices to the soap mixture. This creates interesting colors and textures. Soap-making can be fun. If you keep records of your soap-making recipes, you will be able to recreate a good idea.

To create a wonderful gift for yourself or others, put together a basket with homemade soap, a bath salt or oil mixture, and then add a luffa sponge that you have grown yourself. Sources to purchase the seeds for luffa sponges are as close as your favorite seed company or store.

Luffas are a relative of the squash family and would need a trellis to climb on. The fruit is fast-growing and great to use. Right before the autumn rains start, bring the luffa indoors to dry. You might want to wipe the outer gourd with a weak bleach solution to keep black spots from forming on the outer shell. When completely dry, soak the gourd in warm water overnight so the shell will be easy to peel away. If you wish to whiten the fiber of the sponge, soak the gourd in a weak bleach solution. This will also soften the outer shell.

To soften the sponges, use them for household tasks, such as wiping down counter tops or scrubbing out sinks. When the sponge has been softened by this hard work, it will be soft enough to use for your bath. These sponges last forever and you need never buy another sponge. They are a handy gift from Mother Nature, if we but take the time to plant them.

EASY HERBAL SOAP: Place 2 tablespoons finely chopped lemon verbena or lavender into 2 tablespoons warmed glycerin. Place in a warm area for several days. Strain and finely grate 12 tablespoons of unscented soap or soap flakes and melt in top of a double boiler. Remove from heat and add the scented glycerin to the melted soap. Add 1 tablespoon of honey. Mix well. Pour into greased molds. Allow to set until the soap is cool and hardened.

Now that we've taken the steps needed to care for our skin properly, here are some recipes that will take care of special problems and needs.

CHAPPED SKIN: Children and adults who spend a lot of time outdoors can be prone to chapped hands. Make a tea, pouring 1 pint boiling water over 2 tablespoons dried chamomile. Let steep overnight. Strain and refrigerate. Use on face and hands as you would a lotion.

CHAPPED SKIN: Pour 1 pint boiling water over 5 tablespoons of calendula petals. Let steep 30 minutes. Strain and use as a compress. Very soothing. Also good for minor cuts and scrapes.

SKIN INFECTIONS: Pour 1 cup of baking soda in your bath water and soak for 15 minutes. Baking soda helps to balance the P.H. of your skin and allows it to heal naturally.

LESSENS REDNESS OF SKIN: Cover a handful of parsley with mineral water. Soak 24 hours. Strain. Apply to face as a rinse.

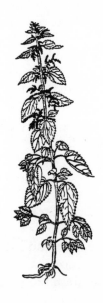

Common Nettle (Urtica dioica)

NETTLE RASH: Nettle rash can be very painful. The juice of nettle will neutralize it's own sting. Apply as a tea. This tea is also good to treat sunburn. Put 1 teaspoon of dried nettle in 1 cup of boiling water. Remove from heat. Cover and steep until cooled. Strain. Apply freely on sunburn or nettle rash.

NETTLE RASH: Rub the leaves of mullein on the nettle rash to remove the discomfort and pain from the rash. Crush the leaves until juicy and rub on the rash. This should provide immediate relief.

I have a patch of nettle near my house and my grandchildren have been in contact with it several times. I found several plants of mullein that I could transplant close to the house so I would have it handy for any nettle rashes. It does not transplant very easily, so you may have to try several times. Try to find plants that grow in soil similar to your soil. I know for a fact it will not live if transplanted from soil that is totally different from the area you plan to move it to. Mullein is handy for many different treatments, so even if you are not close to nettle, there are many other ways in which to use it. It is an attractive plant. Sometimes it can reach majestic heights of 6 feet or more, with yellow blooms that are refreshing to see.

POISON IVY: Cut open a green tomato and squeeze the juice on the area affected. This works if you use the juice as soon as you come into contact with the poison ivy. Rinse the area immediately with water, than apply the juice from the tomato.

POISON IVY TREATMENT: Mix equal parts of buttermilk, vinegar, and salt. Rub on the affected area. Use this after the rash has appeared. Helps stop the itching and soothes the area. I do not get poison ivy, but have used it on friends and family with success.

POISON IVY: Put 1 quart of willow leaves in 1 quart of water. Boil for 15 minutes. Strain and cool. The liquid should turn a dark brown. If it doesn't, let it sit until color comes. Rub on the affected area after it cools.

POISON IVY: Apply paste of baking soda and water to the affected area liberally. This will stop itching. This works as good as calamine lotion.

POISON OAK: If possible, apply the juice from crushed jewel-weed stems to the area immediately. Also, you can put a large handful of jewelweed into 2 pints of water and boil for 15 minutes. Strain and apply to the area affected. We have poison oak in our woods, so I have several jewelweed plants that I plan to transplant to use for remedies. We are putting in an acre pond and the jewel-weed is growing right where the pond will be. I would still try to save the plants even if I did not have a use for them as they are attractive and interesting plants.

EMERGENCY SKIN ERUPTION: This is good for teenagers to use. Steep 2 papaya mint tea bags in 1/2 cup of boiling water. Let sit until tea is very strong. Heat to a degree that is bearable to skin and apply as a compress to the eruption. This does help. I know because many of my younger friends have tried it with success. Teenage girls swear by it.

FACIEI SEBORRHEA: Faciei seborrhea is a condition resulting from a functional disease of the sebaceous glands, which cause an increase in the amount of sebaceous secretion. It can cause elevat-ed patches with red borders, covered with scars and crusts. Con-sult with your physician for treatment if severe. He or she would probably want you to use a hydrocortisone cream. If the scalp is affected, use a shampoo that contains selenium sulfide or sulfur. If the condition is not too severe, apply apple cider vinegar directly to the face daily for 10-15 days.

ECZEMA TREATMENT: Eczema can be caused by an allergic reaction. The cause is a combination of external as well as internal conditions. No class, age or sex is exempt. It can be brought on by contact with certain chemicals. A balanced natural diet plays a large part in treating eczema.If you suffer from eczema, look care-fully at your eating habits and the chemicals you ingest daily, either through the skin or digestion. The condition can be caused by psychological factors and stress can make the condition worse. Heartsease is one treatment that has been used by Native Ameri-cans for centuries. Add 2 tablespoons of heartsease (pansy) in 2 cups boiling water. Steep until cool. Use as wash.

Another treatment that seems to work is to use tincture of valerian. I have had some success with certain people using the valerian tincture applied with a cotton ball and allowing it to dry naturally. The recipe for making the tincture is in chapter eleven. I use this tincture to successfully treat many itching and scaling skin conditions. Most people do not like the smell of valerian, but if it works, who cares?

ECZEMA TREATMENT: Grate a raw potato and use as a poultice to relieve the itching. Apply as a poultice. This is good to use for instant relief from itching.

RASHES AND ECZEMA: The leaves of sheep sorrel (*rumex acetosella*) are good in curing disorders such as rashes and eczema. Pound a handful of the leaves and apply as a poultice.

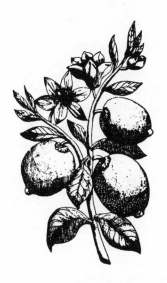

Lemon (Citrus limon)

ECZEMA TREATMENT: Apply lemon juice to the area and allow to dry before bed. Leave on overnight. Helps the skin to heal. This can dry the area and promote healing. It acts as an antiseptic if the area is inflamed.

Many times you may be using a remedy that you may not think is classified as an herb. But every tree, plant or flower is an herb. The by-product of a lemon tree is a lemon and is therefore classified as an herb. Any natural remedy that comes from a tree, flower, shrub, vine, or spice is considered an herbal remedy.

SKIN RASH: Add 1 cup of red clover blossoms and leaves to 2 cups of boiling water. Allow to steep until cool. Strain and apply to skin rash and allow to dry naturally. Reapply as often as needed.

HEAT RASH: Combine 1 ounce each of powdered chamomile and powdered calendula. Add 1/2 ounce of corn starch. Mix well and use to soothe heat rash.

DIAPER RASH: Diaper rash can be caused by too much acid in the system. Give the child plenty of water and try giving cranberry juice in the bottle. Kids love it and it does neutralize the acids in urine.

Also, external factors such as laundry soap may cause a severe diaper rash. Try washing the diapers in a mild homemade lye soap. I know that disposable diapers are the easiest to use, but please give consideration to the environment before making a decision to use them. Perhaps you could use them for outings only and use cloth diapers at home.

If diaper rash is already evident, try this lotion to soothe baby and speed healing. Pour 1 cup of boiling water over 1 tablespoon chamomile. Let steep, covered, until cool. Strain and add 2 tablespoons cod-liver oil to the herb water. Shake well and apply to diaper rash after gently washing the area.

CRADLE CAP AND DIAPER RASH: Cradle cap is a seborrheic dermatitis of the scalp that causes lesions of the scalp and sometimes the face. Shampoo daily, using a mild natural shampoo. Prepare the following rinse and use it after shampooing. Put 1/2 cup of calendula and 1/2 cup chamomile flowers in 1 pint of boiling water. Let steep for 30 minutes. Strain and use as a rinse after shampooing. Leftover liquid can be added to the bath water. It's very soothing and helps to control cradle cap. Make sure the baby drinks plenty of water as this helps to keep the system flushed of toxins and also helps to clear cradle cap.

IMPETIGO: Children are highly susceptible because impetigo is very contagious. It is caused by a bacterial infection—staphylococcal or streptococcal—or a combination of the two infections. Generally it appears around the nose or mouth. Make sure that you keep the area as dry and clean as possible. Be careful when you are cleaning the area because it is very contagious. Keep away from other children until the lesions are healed. If the area is kept clean, there should be no secondary infections. Split open a leaf of aloe vera and apply the gel directly to the areas affected. Repeat often and keep the area clean.

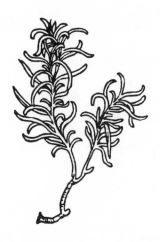

Rosemary (Rosemarinas officinalis)

IMPETIGO TREATMENT: Put 1/4 cup of rosemary leaves and 1/4 cup of thyme in 1 pint of water. Simmer for 15 minutes. Strain, cool and use to clean the area several times daily. Make fresh daily. Use cotton balls to clean the area and dispose of the cotton balls after use. This is a good astringent to use as a wash.

IMPETIGO TREATMENT: This is also good to treat ringworm. Mash a handful of mulberries. Place on area needed and bandage. Mulberries act as an astringent and are good for the treatment of impetigo.

IMPETIGO TREATMENT: Mix 1 cup of water with apple cider vinegar. Use as a wash for impetigo. This may burn if the lesions are open, but it will help to heal the sores.

PSORIASIS: Psoriasis is genetically determined and consists of reddish lesions that have characteristic silvery scaling. The lesions may come and go but generally are chronic. There is a specific type of arthritis that is associated with psoriasis. Check with your physician for treatment if the condition is severe. For home treatment of the scaling and itching of psoriasis, split open an aloe vera leaf and rub on the area affected. The skin absorbs the gel rapidly, so apply plenty and apply often. This stops the itching, and if used regularly seems to help psoriasis. It's also good to use for sunburn. You can purchase aloe gel juice by the gallon and you may want to use the juice as a daily lotion to help control psoriasis.

PSORIASIS: Try using oil of avocado rubbed sparingly on affected areas. It works for quite a few people.

PSORIASIS TREATMENT: Place 1 cup burdock root in 1 pint water and bring to a boil. Reduce heat and simmer for 30 minutes. Strain and apply to the affected area several times daily and you should see results.

TREATMENT FOR SCALY SKIN: Mix together 2 ounces each of lemongrass, rose petals, and corn meal. Add to 2 ounces of witch hazel. Add 1 ounce of the mixture to 1 quart of boiling water. Steep for 30 minutes. Add to bath water. Soak in bath 10-15 minutes.

BURNS: Make a salve using 1 cup solid vegetable shortening, 1/2 ounce beeswax, 1 ounce of Irish moss, 1 ounce white oak bark, 1 ounce marsh mallow root and simmer for 15 minutes. Strain immediately and keep stirring while the mixture is cooling. Add several drops of tincture of benzoin to the salve. This keeps the salve free of bacteria. Where burns are concerned you need to keep the area as clean as possible to prevent infection and permanent scarring. Apply the salve directly to the burned area.

BURNS: Cut open the leaf of aloe vera and apply immediately after a burn occurs, to relieve the pain and prevent scarring.

BURN TREATMENT: Scrape a raw potato and apply to the burn. Reapply as the potato dries. This tends to start cooling the burn immediately. Get help if burn is severe. Until help arrives, you can use the potato to cool the burn.

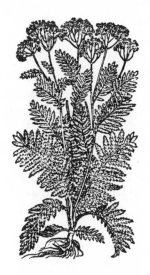

Yarrow (Achillea millefolium)

BURN TREATMENT: Grind up the whole plant of white yarrow. Place in pan and cover with cold water. Allow to steep for several hours. Use this to cool the burn and aid healing.

BURN TREATMENT: Yogurt relieves the pain of a burn fast. Apply to the burned area as soon as possible to relieve the pain.

BURN TREATMENT: Put the burned area in apple cider vinegar if possible. After soaking until the pain is relieved, you may apply a loose bandage that has been soaked in vinegar. Prevents scars and speeds healing as well as relieving pain.

BURN TREATMENT: Put 2 tablespoons of St. John's wort in 1 cup of boiling water. Allow to steep until cool. Strain. Apply as a wash to the burn to relieve pain and speed healing.

BURN TREATMENT: After cooling the burn with cold water, add a paste of apple butter. Reapply as the apple butter dries. Keeps the burn from leaving a scar and promotes healing.

TREATING FROSTBITE: Put 1/4 ounce of alum in a pan of hot water. Soak the hands or feet in the liquid for 15 minutes. Cover with socks or gloves to keep warm.

TREATING FROSTBITE: Massage kerosene on the parts affected. Then apply warmed olive oil and keep warm. Give a warm cinnamon tea or any that is a stimulant. 1 teaspoon of cayenne pepper added to 1 cup of warm water is good to stimulate circulation. Drink several cups about an hour apart.

SORES THAT WON'T HEAL: Boil a small handful of elder leaves in 2 cups of milk until the leaves are soft. Strain off the leaves and return milk to a boil until the herb mixture thickens. Apply as a wash on the hard-to-heal sore or wound. Repeat frequently until wound loses that angry look. I have had several friends report that this is a great remedy for open ulcers on the legs that are hard to heal. *Please note: sometimes these sores are warning signs of a more serious condition. Don't hesitate to consult your doctor.*

TREAT BOILS OR SORES: It has been my belief that boils are caused by blood impurities and certain minerals missing from the diet. If you are prone to boils, look at your diet and take steps to remedy that. It is important that you have a good balanced diet that includes plenty of vegetables. Plenty of water daily aids the body in flushing toxins from your system. Try mixing equal parts of cayenne pepper, powdered lecithin, butchers broom, and apple pectin and placing in #00 capsules. Take 2 daily along with a multiple B vitamin tablet to improve circulation and flush the body of toxins. To help heal a boil or sore, hold a plantain leaf under very hot running water. Crush the leaf until limp. Place over the inflammation. This is a very good astringent.

BOILS: Native Americans used wild pansy (heartsease) to draw boils. It was ground up and placed on the boil, bandaged and left on overnight.

SOFTEN BOILS: Apply linseed oil to the boil to soften and aid in healing.

BOILS: To bring a boil to a head, place a small piece of fatty bacon over the boil and bandage it. Leave on overnight. Should be ready to remove the head by the next morning.

BOILS: Take a handful of crushed parsley and wrap in cheesecloth. Apply to the boil and wrap a hot cloth around the area. Repeat, covering the area with the hot cloth for about 15 minutes.

BOILS: Soak a piece of bread in lemon juice and apply to the boil. Cover with a loose bandage and try to leave on overnight.

SHINGLES: Shingles can be a very serious disorder. It is an eruption of acute, inflammatory, herpetic vesicles along a peripheral nerve. You should seek help from your physician, as it can be very painful. Until you are able to reach help, try this to relieve the pain. It really works. Crush 2 aspirins and add 2 tablespoons of clear nail polish. Apply to the affected area. Will give up to 10 hours relief.

SHINGLES: Aloe vera leaf, applied to the area and repeated often, along with 500 mg of vitamin C given every hour, will help. Could take 5-6 hours to obtain relief. Continue treatment until shingles are gone.

INSECT STINGS AND BITES: Rub the area affected with the juice from a honeysuckle vine.

BEE STINGS AND INSECT BITES: Bruise fresh basil leaves and apply directly to the insect sting or bite. I have to use this on my husband quite a bit. For some reason, bees just do not like him. This could be because he does not have good feelings toward them. I have been stung by accidentally stepping on a bee only twice in my life and I guarantee this worked for both of us. It takes a very short time to relieve the pain and reduces swelling. It also stops the itching that often occurs when a sting is healing. Really, you could use any plant that bees are attracted to as an antidote for bee stings. Basil seems to work best for us.

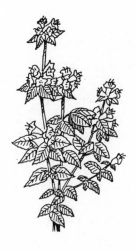

Basil (Ocimum basilicum)

INSECT BITES: Apply fresh crushed parsley directly to the insect bite. It neutralizes the poison and stops the pain.

MOSQUITO BITES: Itching should stop immediately if you apply table salt to the moistened area. You can help to control the population of mosquitoes by keeping the area around your home clean. Get rid of any open containers that hold water. They become quite prolific if allowed a place to propagate. Prevention is the better policy. Apply pennyroyal oil if you are in an area where there is a large population of mosquitoes. This keeps them away.

INSECT BITES: Apply spirits of ammonia to the bite. Should relieve itching immediately.

SPIDER BITES: Apply equal parts salt and baking soda mixed with enough water to make a paste. Apply to the spider bite. Will relieve the pain and itching.

INSECT BITES: Make a paste of commercial meat tenderizer and place on bite. Neutralizes the poison in just a few minutes.

INSECT BITES: Apply a dab of toothpaste to the area. Stops itching fast.

INSECT BITES: Mix PABA with alcohol and apply to the swollen area. Swellings disappear overnight.

INSECT BITE PREVENTIVE: Before going to an area that you know has many insects, take 1 tablet of 100 mg thiamine. If you are going to be out several days, hiking or camping, take several tablets a day. Insects stay away.

SUNBURN: Apply vinegar directly to the sunburn. Relieves pain quickly. Make several applications and apply as soon as possible.

SUNBURN: Taking a PABA tablet of at least 100 mg a day should stop you from burning. Apply PABA lotion also.

TO REMOVE WARTS: My father had the gift of rubbing warts to make them go away overnight. I well remember people coming to him to have their warts rubbed. I honestly can't remember one time where it failed. Several people have mentioned that rubbing castor oil on the warts also help to dispel them.

WART REMOVER: Apply the milk from a dandelion stem several times daily. This is said to work well.

WART REMOVER: Rubbing the milk from milkweed several times daily also is good to use. This was a popular remedy used by Native Americans.

WART REMOVER: Apply warm castor oil to a bandage and apply to the wart. Replace 3 times a day until wart dissolves. It shouldn't take more than a week.

WART REMOVER: Apply the juice of a cashew nut directly on the wart and bandage. Reapply several times daily.

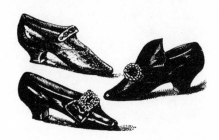

TO REMOVE CORNS: Corns are caused by ill-fitting shoes. It really is good to go barefoot as much as possible. I think the Asian practice of removing shoes as you enter a house is an excellent habit. I always allowed my children to go barefoot indoors and outdoors as much as possible while their feet were forming. None of them have foot problems. They seemed to learn to walk earlier and have stronger foot and leg muscles. I never wear shoes unless I have to. Besides being good for my feet, it feels so good!

If you are diabetic you need to seek help from your physician immediately for any foot problem and that is the one exception I make to going barefoot. Diabetics should wear shoes at all times to protect their feet from accidental cuts.

If you already suffer from corns, try these remedies to get rid of them and then make a practice of going barefoot and getting proper-fitting shoes. It may cost a little more, but your health is your most important asset you have. Soak bruised ivy leaves in vinegar overnight. Soak a small piece of bread in the vinegar mixture and apply to corn. Bind up and leave on during the day. Replace with fresh application at night. Continue treatment until corn is gone.

CORN TREATMENT: Remove soft corns by dipping a clean cloth in turpentine and wrapping it around the area. Continue treatment until the corn is gone. Apply turpentine a couple times a day by pouring it on the cloth.

CORN TREATMENT: Bind a fresh lemon slice to the corn and leave on overnight. Soaking the feet in baking soda and water will also dissolve the corn.

CORN TREATMENT: Place a slice of raw onion over the corn each night and bandage. Removes the corn in 3-4 weeks. Pulverized garlic cloves will also work.

TREAT OR PREVENT ATHLETE'S FOOT: Athlete's foot is caused by a fungus infection of the outer "dead" layer of the skin. Prevention is the best treatment. Careful attention to hygiene is important. Ventilation of the feet is very important. Going barefoot a lot at home helps the feet to stay dry. When going into public showers or pool areas, wear thongs to prevent infection. When you do wear shoes, lightly dust the feet and shoes with powdered alum to prevent moisture. Wear cotton socks to absorb moisture.

ATHLETE FEET TREATMENT: Put 2 tablespoons of red clover in 1/2 cup of boiling water. Steep until cool. Add enough corn starch to make a paste. Spread this paste on feet and put socks on. Leave the paste on overnight.

REMEDY FOR ATHLETE'S FOOT: Flower of sulfur can be dusted on the feet and shoes to treat or prevent the fungi from taking hold. Flower of sulfur can be purchased at your drugstore.

TREATMENT FOR ATHLETE'S FOOT: Add 1/2 cup of sea salt to a basin of very hot water. Soak the feet daily in this mixture for 30 minutes until improvement is noticed.

REMEDY FOR ATHLETE'S FOOT: Put plenty of apple cider vinegar all over the feet. Soak a cotton ball in the vinegar and place these between the toes. Put on socks and leave on overnight.

REMEDY FOR ATHLETE'S FEET: Rub lemon juice on the feet and allow to dry. Try to go barefoot as much as possible. Reapply the lemon juice several times daily.

REMEDY FOR FOOT ODOR: Sprinkle baking soda in your shoes to eliminate odor. Soaking your feet in baking soda and water will eliminate strong odor and is restful for tired feet as well.

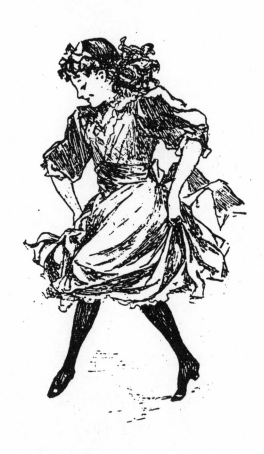

·5·

Colds and Chest Complaints

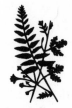

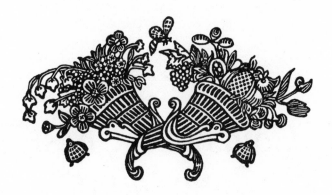

Herbs used for medicinal purposes are made in many different ways. Many times we can use a simple tea to treat an ailment that is not serious enough to seek help from our physician.

PREPARING INFUSIONS AND
DECOCTIONS FOR HOME REMEDIES

When an herbal tea infusion (STEEPED), or decoction (BOILED) is used, it is best taken on an empty or near empty stomach. They are generally taken 1 hour before a meal unless the recipe says differently.

When preparing an infusion, you need to prepare a fresh cup for each dose. Sip the dosage slowly, never gulp it down. You really should swish it around the mouth before swallowing. This helps the liquid to mix with the enzymes in the saliva and rapidly assimilates the herbs into the blood stream. Generally the dosage would be 3-4 cups per day. The herb chosen for an infusion should be allowed to steep for anywhere from 10-25 minutes covered. Strain and drink warm, not hot, unless the recipe tells you to drink the tea hot.

When preparing an infusion, 1 teaspoon of the herb mixture to 1 cup of boiling water is the general recipe. Sometimes the recipes will call for more of the herb. Follow the instructions of each specific recipe because there are exceptions to every rule.

A decoction is a concentrate. The usual recipe for a decoction is 1 tablespoon of the herb's bark or roots to 1 quart of water. The liquid is boiled (covered) until half of it has evaporated. It is then strained and placed in the refrigerator until needed. When preparing a decoction dose, you would add 1-3 tablespoons of the liquid to a cup of warm water. Then it is ready to drink.

Most of the recipes in this chapter are for infusions (teas) but there are some decoctions included.

COLDS, CHEST COMPLAINTS AND ASTHMA

While we all get colds at one time or another, we can minimize the severity and length of the illness by the condition we keep our system in. Some of the herbs we will be using in this chapter are called **expectorants, demulcents,** and **diaphoretics**.

Diaphoretics cause the patient to perspire and increase blood circulation, thus helping the system to get rid of accumulated poisons and toxins in the body.

Expectorants can and do help the body in dispelling mucus from the system.

Demulcents soothe irritated and inflamed areas, thus allowing the body to heal.

Put the patient on a light diet during the illness and while recuperating. If the patient is in a weakened condition, do not use a strong stimulant. Give clear broths and tonics to build the strength back up.

TO STAVE OFF INFECTIONS: Hyssop tea, if used on a regular basis, is said to help keep away infections. Add several teaspoons of the chopped leaves to 2 cups of boiling water and allow to steep 15 minutes. Strain and sweeten with honey. Take several cups per day if fighting a cold or infection.

FEVERFEW BREW: Pour 1 pint boiling water over 1 ounce of dried feverfew flowers. Let steep until cool. Strain and reheat. Drink HOT, sweetened with honey or sugar.

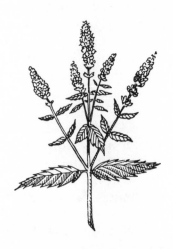

Peppermint (Mentha piperita)

TRADITIONAL PEPPERMINT CURE: Mix 1 tablespoon elder flowers, 1 tablespoon peppermint, 1 tablespoon white yarrow, and 1 tablespoon feverfew. Pour 2 cups boiling water over the herb mix. Cover and let steep for 15 minutes. Strain, sweeten and drink hot. This recipe helps to break a fever by causing the patient to perspire. The yarrow acts as a pain reliever and makes the patient more comfortable. If the cold is not severe, you need add only 1 teaspoon of the herb mixture to 1 cup of boiling water. Eases the patient and helps to dispel mucus.

COLD TREATMENT: At the onset of a cold, add 1/2 teaspoon each of cinnamon and ginger to 1 cup of scalded milk. Add 1 tablespoon of honey and drink while hot. Very soothing and stimulating.

COLD TREATMENT: Mullein flower tea has a pleasant taste and is good to soothe inflamed conditions of the mucous membrane lining the throat. Also relieves coughing. Put a small handful of the mullein flowers in 1 pint of boiling water. Allow to steep 15 minutes. Strain and sweeten with honey.

COLD TREATMENT: Chop several leaves of comfrey and add 1/2 cup of elderberries. Add 1 cup of honey and 1 cup of water.

Simmer for 30 minutes. Strain and take as needed to produce perspiration and reduce fever. The comfrey leaves produce an aspirin-like substance and help to ease the discomforts of a cold, as well as soothe inflamed mucous membranes of the throat. Comfrey is considered a demulcent, and an expectorant. The elderberries serve as a diuretic to flush the system.

COLD TREATMENT: Heat a glass of lemonade and add honey to sweeten. This is a good recipe if you have a cold with a fever. It relaxes you and is helpful in relieving discomfort.

ROYAL MIX FOR SEVERE COLDS: Mix 1 cup each of dried white yarrow, spearmint, sage, catnip, horehound, verbena and pennyroyal. Pour 1 pint of boiling water over 2-1/2 tablespoons of the herb mix. Cover and let stand 10 minutes. Strain and sweeten. Reheat and drink 1 cup every couple of hours. Use more often if sweating is desired.

CINNAMON TEA: This is really good to take during a cold, as it will cause you to sweat. Cinnamon is a strong stimulant and this really works. Simmer 6 sticks of cinnamon in 1 pint of water for 30 minutes. Strain and add milk and honey after removing the cinnamon sticks. Tastes delicious and kids love it.

RICE TEA: This is another tea that kids and grownups both love. Simmer 1/2 cup of rice in 1-1/2 quarts of water for 15 minutes. Strain and add a few drops of vanilla flavoring and sugar. Sprinkle with cinnamon for extra flavor. Drink warm. This settles an upset stomach quickly. This is really good to stop vomiting or diarrhea fast. Rice tea really soothes the stomach and helps the patient get needed rest. This tea is a favorite of mine and it is good to drink simply because you like it. Very nutritious.

ROSEHIP TEA: Pour 1 cup boiling water over 1 teaspoon of crushed rosehips and 1 teaspoon of dried lemon peel. Let steep 15 minutes. Strain and use honey to sweeten. Drink this tea whether you have a cold or not. The extra vitamin C is good for you anytime.

COLD TREATMENT: Boil 8 cornhusks in 2 pints of water for about 30 minutes. Strain and drink. Said to relieve headaches and stuffiness of the nose during a cold.

FOOT BATHS FOR COLDS: Put 1/2 pound of dried mustard in 2 quarts of boiling water and boil for 10 minutes. Add this liquid to foot bath to treat colds and respiratory problems.

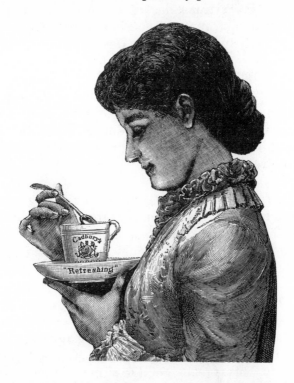

COLD REMEDY: Put 1 gallon of water in a large pan, adding 3 ounces softened ginger root, 3 cups of honey, and 1/4 pound seedless raisins. Bring to a boil and simmer for about an hour. The top will have to be skimmed every once in a while. Cool, strain and place in a tightly closed container overnight in the refrigerator. The next day, squeeze 6 lemons and 4 oranges and add to the mixture. Mix well and drink 2-3 glasses per day. This will get rid of symptoms pretty fast and clean the system.

COLDS WITH FEVER: Steep 1 teaspoon of catnip in 1 cup boiling water for 10 minutes. Strain and add the tea to 1 cup of cherry juice. Catnip has been used since antiquity to reduce fever by causing the patient to perspire.

SWEETEN BREATH DURING COLDS: Chew fresh parsley during a cold. This not only freshens the breath during a cold, but rids the mouth of any bad odors anytime. Parsley also gives you the extra vitamins you need while suffering through a cold.

FEVER WITH COLDS: Take 1 ounce of elder flowers or white yarrow and add 1 ounce of peppermint leaves. Simmer the leaves in 1 pint of water for 30 minutes. Strain and drink by the 1/2 cupful during the day, as long as fever is present.

COLDS WITH FLU SYMPTOMS: Mix 1 cup each of plantain, black elder flowers, juniper berries, rosemary, Irish moss and peppermint. Steep 1 teaspoon of the herb mix in 1 cup boiling water for 15 minutes. Strain, reheat and sweeten. Drink twice daily.

FLU SYMPTOMS: Pour 2 quarts boiling water over 1 ounce of dried sage. Add the juice of 1 lemon, 1 orange, and 1 ounce of honey. Mix well, cover and steep for 1 hour. Strain and drink as often as desired. Reheat as needed.

FLU REMEDY: Pour 2 pints of boiling water over 1 ounce of elder flowers and 1 ounce of peppermint leaves. Cover and let steep 15 minutes. Strain and sweeten. Give 1 cup warm every hour to produce sweating.

FOR FLU: Put 1 tablespoon each of white yarrow, boneset, and skullcap in a pint of water. Simmer for 30 minutes. Strain. Add 1 tablespoon of this liquid and 1 teaspoon of psyllium seed, flavored, to one cup of boiling water. Sweeten with corn syrup. Drink every 30 minutes. This takes care of backaches and headaches too.

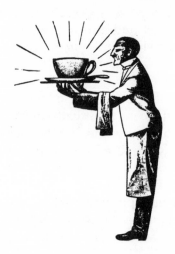

CONGESTIONS WITH COLD: If congestion is present, try this comfrey recipe. Add 1 ounce of comfrey root (cut up fine) to 1 pint of water. Bring to a boil and then simmer for 30 minutes. Strain and sweeten. Take this 3-4 times daily by the cup. Comfrey reduces the inflammation in the the bronchial and alimentary system. It acts as an emollient, demulcent and expectorant. Not bad for one simple herb. It also has pain-relieving properties, so you are more comfortable while fighting a cold.

FOR CHEST CONGESTION, USE THIS OLD INDIAN METHOD: Lightly fry onions and place in a flannel cloth. Add spirit of camphor if you have it. Lightly grease chest with olive oil and place the onion poultice to the chest area and cover to keep warm. My sister had frequent chest problems and this was used by my parents throughout her childhood. It always helped.

CHEST CONGESTION: Mix equal parts ground mustard with flour (half and half). Moisten with tepid water to the consistency of a paste. Spread on muslin cloth. Lightly grease chest area with olive oil and apply this poultice to the chest. Cover with a flannel cloth to keep warm. Leave the poultice on for about 15 minutes or until the skin reddens. Do not allow the poultice to stay on the chest over the amount of time stated.

Caution: You need to apply olive oil to the chest before applying any of the poultices. This protects the skin from burns. The mustard could possibly cause blisters to form if the area is not protected by the olive oil, or if the poultice is left on for too long.

MUSTARD PLASTER: Add enough water to 1/2 cup dry mustard to make a paste. Beat 1-2 egg whites and fold them into the mustard paste. Spread a thin layer of this mixture onto a warm and damp flannel cloth. Rub the chest area with olive oil and apply the plaster. Cover to keep the area warm. Remove when the skin starts to redden.

CHEST CONGESTION: This is an old Chinese method of dealing with chest congestion. Slice and roast several large onions. Pour enough vegetable oil or melted lard over the onions to cover them, and allow to steep in the oven for 30 minutes. Put the onion mixture on a flannel cloth. Grease chest with olive oil and apply the onion poultice to the chest. Cover to keep the poultice warm. Remove after about 30 minutes.

CHEST CONGESTION: Mix 1/2 cup each of powdered slippery elm, corn starch, and crushed black mustard seed. Wet the mixture just enough to make a thin paste. Grease the chest with olive oil. Place the mixture on a warm flannel cloth and apply to the chest. Cover to keep warm. Keep on until chest skin begins to redden.

CHEST CONGESTION: Mix together 2 teaspoons cayenne pepper, 4 tablespoons of cinnamon, and 6 tablespoons powdered ginger. Add enough olive or vegetable oil to form a paste. Apply the mixture to a warm flannel cloth. Grease the chest area with olive oil and apply the poultice to the chest. Cover to keep warm and leave on overnight. All the ingredients are great stimulants and will cause the patient to perspire.

CONGESTION TREATMENT: Mix 1 cup warm almond oil with 1/2 teaspoon of peppermint oil. Massage the chest and back to relieve chest congestion. Keep warm and give plenty of peppermint tea to produce sweating. This works very well. My sister uses this recipe to treat her children when they have chest congestion.

LEMON JUICE AS AN AID: Lemon juice can be added to the herbal teas. It does have a lot of vitamin C and helps to cut through congestion and mucus. I always add lemon juice to my teas. I figure a little extra help doesn't hurt. Lemon juice is also a great astringent and I figure this helps too.

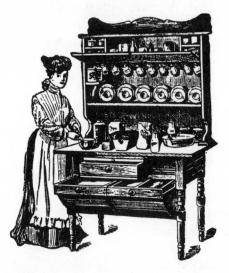

BRONCHITIS TREATMENT: Bronchitis is an inflammation of the mucous membrane of the bronchial tubes. Some people are more prone to infection here then others. The infection is often preceded by a common cold, flu, or can be caused by a streptococcus organism. The predisposing factors may be chilling, fatigue, or even malnutrition. Many times the predisposition can be attributed to allergies or inhalation of chemical agents such as fumes or dust particles.

Treatment of chronic bronchitis should be supervised by your family physician. He or she will find the reason that you suffer from chronic bronchitis and treat you accordingly. Your treatment may require a change in living habits. Smokers have to stop smoking. You may even have to change your sleeping habits. Never sleep in an extremely cold room and be sure to cover your mouth during very cold weather when outdoors. Bed rest is advised along with plenty of fluids and a light diet. Broths, fruit juices, and again, I stress plenty of water.

Allergy related bronchitis is best treated with bee pollen. One teaspoon of pollen granules should be taken daily. During an attack, Vitamin C should be taken in doses of 1000 mg every hour. Vitamin C has an anti-infection action and will help the immune system to regain balance, enabling it to fight the infection.

BRONCHITIS TREATMENT: Mix together 1/2 cup of castor oil and 1/4 cup of turpentine. Warm it before rubbing on the chest at bedtime. Cover with a flannel cloth to keep the area warm. Drink plenty of fluids.

BRONCHITIS POULTICE: Fry onions and apply to the chest after rubbing the chest area with olive oil. Cover with a flannel cloth to keep the area warm. Place a hot water bottle over the chest area to break the congestion fast.

BRONCHITIS TREATMENT: Pour 1 can of asparagus in the blender. Liquefy and refrigerate. Drink 1/4 cup every morning and before retiring to bed. Add water to make a hot drink if desired. You should notice quite an improvement in chronic bronchitis in a few weeks.

BRONCHIAL PROBLEMS: Heat 1 cup of milk, add 1 tablespoon dried bee balm to the milk, and allow to steep 15 minutes. Strain and reheat. Drink several glasses a day until improvement is noticed.

COMFREY BRONCHIAL INFUSION: Put 1/4 ounce of comfrey leaves in 1 pint of boiling water. Cover and steep (covered) 30 minutes. Strain and sweeten with honey. Drink at least 2 cups per day.

BRONCHIAL COUGH: Mix 1 tablespoon of Irish moss, 1 tablespoon comfrey, 1 tablespoon lobelia, 1 tablespoon wild cherry bark, 1 tablespoon verbena, and 1 tablespoon aniseed in 1 pint of water. Boil down to half the liquid. Strain and add 1 pint of honey. Bring to a boil again, then lower heat to simmer for 10 minutes. Remove from heat and add 3 tablespoons of raspberry vinegar before mixing well and storing in the refrigerator. Take 1 tablespoon as needed for cough.

PARSLEY COUGH TREATMENT: This is good to use for a persistent stubborn cough. Pour 2-1/2 cups of boiling water over 2 tablespoons of dried agrimony flowers or leaves, and 1 tablespoon dried parsley. Cover and steep until the mixture is cool. Strain. Use as a gargle to soothe sore throats. To stop persistent coughs, take 2-3 tablespoons of the infusion morning and evening.

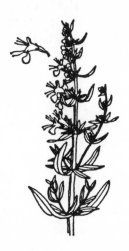

Hyssop (Hyssopus officinalis)

HYSSOP TREATMENT: Hyssop leaves are used to grow the mold that produces penicillin. The tea made from hyssop is very good to treat colds and congestion. Licorice mint (anise hyssop), a member of the hyssop family, makes a very pleasant tea to drink as it has a light licorice taste. My husband drinks this tea year round, as it is his favorite. In fact, I have to make it every couple of days for him. Add 2-3 tablespoons of the herb to a teapot. Add grated orange and lemon rind to the pot if desired. Pour boiling water over the herb and steep 10-15 minutes. Sweeten and drink hot. Will induce sweating and reduce fever fast.

FEVERS: Fill #00 capsules with cayenne pepper and take 2 capsules every 4 hours. Will cause perspiration and bring down a fever fast. This is a really good herb for helping the circulation and ridding the body of toxins fast.

REDUCE FEVER: This is another way to use pepper to bring down a fever fast. Soak several pods of cayenne pepper in 1 cup of hot water for 30 minutes. After straining, add about 1/4 cup of sugar. Add the juice of 2 oranges and drink hot. This works very well. I know, because I have used this for years.

TO INDUCE SWEATING: Mix 1 tablespoon each of white yarrow, boneset, catnip, thyme, mint of any kind, sage, and verbena. If you would like to substitute any of those herbs, use linden, elder flowers, pennyroyal, or horehound. Steep 1 heaping teaspoon of the herbal mixture in 1 cup boiling water for 10 minutes. Strain and sweeten. Drink warm every 3-4 hours. If profuse sweating is desired, drink every hour.

BEST FOR BRINGING OUT MEASLES, AS IT WILL INDUCE SWEATING: Measles is a childhood disease that was thought at one time to be an uncomplicated disease. We now know that complications can and do happen. Best treatment is to have the little patient stay in bed and keep the room dimly lit. Provide quiet activities to keep the patient as quiet as possible. Provide plenty of liquids and keep the patient on a light, wholesome diet. Tepid baths seem to help the patient keep fever down and provide comfort. If the child is running a fever and the rash has not yet broken out, this herbal remedy will help them. Once the rash has broken out, the fever seems to go down somewhat. The disease lasts about 5 days. The fever should subside during those 5 days as the rash starts to disappear.

To prepare the herbal remedy, pour 3 cups boiling water over 1 tablespoon of calendula flowers. Steep 15 minutes. Strain and flavor with 1 drop of peppermint oil and sweeten with sugar. Drink hot, one cup per day.

TREATING PNEUMONIA: Pneumonia is an is an inflammation of the lungs and is caused primarily by bacteria, viruses and chemical irritants. There are really more then 50 causes and it would be too lengthy to go into here. *Caution:* A physician should be consulted because there are complications from pneumonia.

If you are unable to seek medical help, there are ways you can deal with it until medical help is reached. Symptoms begin suddenly and include chills and high fever, cough and sometimes bloody sputum. There is often pain in the chest. I have had what they call "walking pneumonia" and I can tell you it is nothing to fool around with. The mortality rate is high without proper treatment. These are ways to treat pneumonia until you have reached a physician.

Place macerated garlic cloves in a pan and cover with water. Bring the liquid to a boil. Allow fumes to be very strong. If possible, have the patient in the room while you are cooking the garlic. Place a cloth in the liquid and apply the cloth to the chest area. Remove when cool and reheat the cloth by dipping again into the garlic water. Keep this treatment up. Place some of the garlic from the mixture into a quart jar and cover with boiling oil, and keep the container tightly closed to retain the strength while not in use. Have the patient inhale the fumes from the jar while you are replacing the hot cloth. If the patient is able, have them eat small pieces of garlic during treatment.

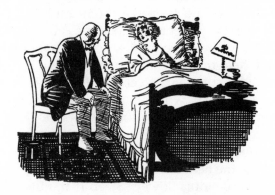

PLEURISY: Pleurisy is an inflammation of the pleura. There is fever and intense sharp pain under the rib cage. Bed rest is a must as is teaching the patient to splint or hold the chest area when coughing. Apply warm or cool compresses to the painful area to decrease inflammation and relieve pain. Give the patient plenty of fluids to help liquify and remove secretions from the system. Have the patient lie on the affected side to prevent transfer of organisms to the unaffected side. A light liquid diet helps in the healing of the patient. Violet tea is very good to treat pleurisy as it has more vitamin A then any known plant. Chop 1 tablespoon of violet leaves, flowers and stems. Pour 1 cup boiling water over the herb and allow to steep (covered) 10 minutes. Strain and sweeten with sugar. Drink as often as desired. Violets are also a great relaxant and this will help to keep the patient calm.

PLEURISY TREATMENT: Mix 1 tablespoon each of ginger, boneset, elecampane, Irish moss, elder flowers, milkweed root and white yarrow. Add 2 tablespoons of the herb mixture to 1 quart of water and boil down to half the liquid. Strain well and add 1 teaspoon oil of peppermint and about 8 ounces of honey. Take 1 tablespoon every 2 hours.

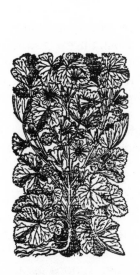 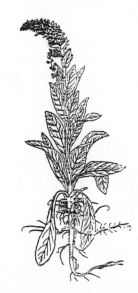

Mallow (Malva sylvestris)   *Mullein (Verbascum rhomifolium)*

EXPECTORANT FOR COUGHS: Mix 1/4 cup each of mullein and mallow flowers. (Either the mullein leaves or flowers can be used.) Add 1 tablespoon of herb mixture to 1 cup of boiling water. Strain and add several cloves and 1 teaspoon of lemon juice. Sweeten with honey. Loosens chest congestion and promotes discharge of mucus.

HOLLYHOCK HELP: This is a good tea for colds and chest complaints. It also soothes the digestive tract. Add 1/4 cup of the chopped leaves and flowers of hollyhock to 1 pint of boiling water. Steep 10 minutes covered. Strain and add honey to sweeten.

WHOOPING COUGH: Whooping cough is an acute infectious disease that is common to children. It causes recurrent spasms of coughing, ending in a whooping inspiration. This recipe works well to suppress the cough.

Squeeze the juice from 3 lemons and mix with 2 beaten egg whites. Add 1/2 cup of brown sugar. Pour 1 small bottle of olive oil in this mixture. Shake well and keep refrigerated. Give 1 teaspoon as needed for cough.

GARLIC COUGH SYRUP: This is a remedy for bronchial complaints ranging from bronchitis to asthma. Slice 1 pound of fresh garlic into 1 quart of water. Bruise 1 ounce each of caraway and fennel seeds. Add to garlic water. Boil this mixture until garlic is soft. Let stand 12-14 hours in a very tightly closed container. Measure the mixture at the end of 14 hours and add equal amount of cider vinegar. Bring again to a boil, adding enough sugar to make a syrup. For coughing, take 1 teaspoon every morning or when necessary.

CHERRY COUGH SYRUP: Place 1 pint of cherries in a pan and add just enough water to cover. Add several lemon slices and 1 pint of honey. Simmer the mixture until cherries are soft. Remove from heat. Remove the lemon slices and the cherry pits from the mixture. Refrigerate and take several tablespoons as needed for coughing.

My grandchildren love this mixture. I have a hard time keeping it on hand, as they take it whether they need it or not. It would also probably be good for someone suffering from gout, as cherries are excellent for treating gout. If you are susceptible to gout, take it on a regular basis to prevent gout attacks.

THYME COUGH SYRUP: Pour 1 pint boiling water over 1 ounce of dried thyme. Cool to room temperature. Strain and add 1 cup of honey. Shake to mix well. Keep refrigerated. Take 1 tablespoon several times a day for sore throats, colds, and coughing.

COUGH SYRUP: Put 1 tablespoon elecampane, 3 tablespoons boneset, 1 tablespoon coltsfoot, 1 tablespoon Irish Moss and 1 tablespoon of lobelia in a pint of water. Boil down to half the liquid. Strain well and add 1 pint of honey. Refrigerate and take by the tablespoon as needed for cough.

COUGH SYRUP: Put 1 tablespoon each of boneset, Irish moss, white yarrow, slippery elm bark, thyme, peppermint, horehound and lemon balm in 1 quart of boiling water. Steep for 30 minutes. Strain well and add 1 quart of honey. Drink several cups of this liquid a day for coughs.

CURRENT COUGH SYRUP: Simmer 3 teaspoons of black currents in 2 cups of water for 15 minutes. Strain and add 2 tablespoons of honey. Use as needed for coughs.

HOREHOUND COUGH SYRUP: Add 3 ounces of horehound and 1 ounce of grated horseradish to 3 cups of water. Bring to a boil and reduce heat to simmer. Simmer until the liquid is reduced by half. Strain and add 3/4 cup of honey. Take 2 teaspoons as needed for coughs.

BORAGE COUGH SYRUP: Place 1/2 cup of borage leaves in blender along with 1/2 cup of water. Blend until mixture is of a smooth consistency. Place in an enamel pan and add 2 cups of honey. Bring to a boil, stirring constantly. Remove from heat and add the juice from 2 lemons. Take 1-2 tablespoons as needed for coughs.

WILD CHERRY COUGH SYRUP: Mix 1 teaspoon each of thyme, lobelia, elecampane, coltsfoot, boneset, mullein, Irish moss, slippery elm bark, wild cherry bark, and 1 tablespoon balm of Gilead. Add mixture to 1 quart of water and simmer until the liquid is reduced by half. Strain and add 1 pint of honey. Add a few drops of wild cherry oil for flavoring. Keep refrigerated after bottling.

Dosage is 1-2 tablespoons for coughing. I keep this handy all the time. It will keep for long periods of time and it does work well.

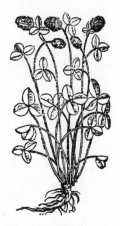

Red Clover (Trifolium pratense)

RED CLOVER COUGH SUPPRESSANT: Place 2 pints of water and 2 pints of honey in pan and bring to a boil. Reduce heat to simmer and add 2 ounces of red clover blossoms. Simmer for 15 minutes. Cool, strain, bottle and refrigerate. Take 1-2 tablespoons as needed for coughs. You receive a lot of extra minerals with this recipe.

ASTHMA: No age is exempt from asthma, although it occurs more frequently in childhood or early adulthood. The wheezing is caused by a spasm of the bronchial tubes or swelling of their mucous membranes. Recurrence and severity of attacks are caused by many different reasons. Mental or physical fatigue; exposure to fumes or chemicals; inhaled allergens; foods; infections of the upper and lower respiratory tracts; and emotional situations can bring on attacks that can last from several hours to several days. Try several of these home treatments to help control asthma attacks.

ASTHMA TREATMENT: If you suffer from asthma, boil some of the aloe vera leaves in a pan of water and inhale the vapors. Put a towel over the head and pan to get the full effects of the vapors.

ASTHMA TREATMENT: Add 1 tablespoon each of coltsfoot, mullein, thyme, and lobelia to 1 pint of water. Simmer at least 1/2 hour, covered. Strain and add 2 cups of honey. Take by the tablespoon until relief is obtained. Flavoring, such as oil of peppermint, may be added if desired.

ASTHMA TREATMENT: Make fresh daily. Cut an onion into very thin slices and place in a bowl. Cover the onion slices with honey and let sit overnight. The next day, scrape the honey from the onion slices and take 1 teaspoon 3-4 times daily.

FENNEL TEA FOR TREATING ASTHMA: Bruise 2 teaspoons of fennel seeds and pour 1 cup of boiling water over the seeds. Allow to steep for 15 minutes covered. Strain and sweeten. If sweetened with sugar, will also aid indigestion.

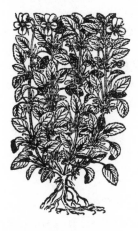

Pansy (Viola tricolor)

PANSY TREATMENT: Pansy is also called heartsease. Tea can be made from the flowers and leaves to treat chronic asthma and to strengthen the heart. It has even been used to treat epilepsy as it an anti-convulsive. Add the chopped leaves and flowers to 1 cup boiling water and steep, covered, for 10 minutes. Strain and sweeten. Drink several cups daily.

ASTHMA TREATMENT: Add several tablespoons of freshly grated horseradish to 1 cup of milk. Simmer for 10 minutes and strain. Drink as necessary to obtain relief.

ASTHMA TREATMENT: Many people drink honeysuckle tea to help with chronic asthma. Put 1 tablespoon of the grated root of honeysuckle in 1 cup of water. Boil gently for 10 minutes. Strain and sweeten. Drink daily.

COFFEE FOR NERVOUS ASTHMA: Coffee is helpful in some forms of asthma. Make the coffee double strength and drink when experiencing difficulties.

ASTHMA: Mix 1 tablespoon each of boneset, Irish moss, coltsfoot, mullein, thyme, rosemary, valerian, and lobelia. Add 1 teaspoon of the herbal mixture to 1 cup of boiling water. Cover and steep for 15 minutes. Strain. Peppermint or cherry oil may be added for flavoring if desired. Drink 4 cups daily to obtain relief.

POTATO TREATMENT FOR ASTHMA: Boil several potatoes. Place in a basin and cover the head and basin with a towel to get the most from the steam.

THYME TREATMENT FOR ASTHMA: Bring to a boil 2 cups of water to which you have added 1 tablespoon of thyme. Pour into a basin and cover head and basin with a towel to inhale the steam.

ASTHMA TINCTURE: Place 2 ounces of lobelia leaves and 2 ounces of lobelia seed (crushed) in 1 pint of raspberry vinegar. Let sit for 2 weeks. Strain and take by the tablespoon during asthma attacks. If needed, take every 10 minutes until relief is obtained. *Caution:* Overdoses of lobelia can cause low blood pressure, respiratory depression, and even coma, followed by death.

To make the raspberry vinegar, mash 2 quarts of fresh or canned raspberries and add to 2 quarts of cider vinegar. Let sit 2 days. Strain. For each quart of liquid add 1 pound of sugar. Bring to a boil, removing the scum as it comes to the top. The longer you boil, the thicker the syrup. You can add this to other cough syrups or teas if desired.

CHERRY TREATMENT FOR ASTHMA: Add a handful of cherry stems to 1 pint of boiling water. Cover and steep until liquid is cool. Strain. Add 1 pint of honey and shake well. Take 1 tablespoon as needed for coughing.

THIS WAS ONCE USED AS A SMOKING TOBACCO FOR ASTHMA: Mix 1 cup each of rosemary, coltsfoot leaves, eyebright, thyme and lavender. Crush and mix well. Roll into cigarettes or place mixture in a pipe for smoking. I don't know anyone who has tried this recipe, but it was said to have been used quite often by Native Americans.

SMOKE TREATMENT: This is said to relieve breathing difficulties. Place dried crushed rosemary in a pipe and smoke for relief.

AIDS BREATHING FOR ASTHMATICS AT BEDTIME: Take 1 tablespoon of sunflower or corn oil before retiring for the night. Helps you to breath easier during the night.

SMOKERS COUGH: Pour 1 cup of boiling water over 1 tablespoon anise seed. Let steep, covered, for 15 minutes. Strain and sweeten with honey. Drink hot.

ASTHMA TREATMENT: Clean the root of mullein very carefully. Add 1 cup of the chopped root to 1 pint of water. Bring to a boil and simmer until the liquid is reduced by half. Strain well and add 1 cup of honey. Give 2 tablespoons as needed. This is also good to use during colds, as it helps to remove phlegm.

CRANBERRY JUICE TREATMENT FOR ASTHMA: Cranberry juice is very good for treating asthma attacks, as it contains an ingredient that dilates the bronchial tubes.

Cook and mash cranberries. Place in a tightly closed glass container and refrigerate. When needed during an attack, add 3 teaspoons of the mashed cranberries to a cup of hot water. Sip while the water is hot.

EMPHYSEMA TREATMENT: Put 6 drops of anise oil in 1 tablespoon of honey. Should take daily after every meal.

WHICH PART OF THE HERB IS USED?

I have listed a few of the herbs that would be used in making some of the recipes. I've also included information on which part of the herb is commonly used to prepare remedies.

ACACIA *(Acacia senegal):* The exudation is the part used. Removes phlegm from the throat and bronchia. Use for conditions of the respiratory and digestive organs.

BLACK ALDER *(Prinos verticillatus):* Bark and fruits are used. Good for treatment of liver and gallbladder problems. Cleans the system of accumulated mucoid toxins.

TAG ALDER *(Alnus serrulata):* Cones and bark are used as a diuretic.

ALKANET *(Alkanna tinctoria):* The root is the part used. Used for blood disorders, liver and gallbladder problems.

✓ **ALLSPICE** *(Lindera benzoin):* Fruit, leaves and twigs are used. Breaks fevers.

ANGELICA *(A. atropurpurea):* Roots, seeds and leaves are used. Expectorant for colds and coughs. Also treats kidney disorders and aids the digestive system.

ANISE *(Pimpinella anisum):* The leaves and seeds are used. Anise is good for colds and flu. Licorice or anise hyssop is a great tea to relieve fever. It is used as a digestive aid. It can be added to recipes for teas which include unpleasant-tasting herbs. Anise adds a nice licorice flavor to any tea.

APPLE *(Pyrus malus):* The whole fruit is used. Dried apple tea is an excellent diuretic. Aids in elimination of toxins from the system.

ASPARAGUS *(Asparagus officinalis):* The shoots and the roots are used. Warm tea made from asparagus is used as an excellent diuretic. Drink every 2-3 hours.

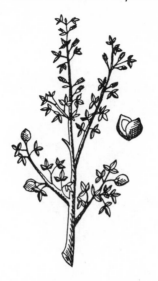

Balm of Gilead (Populus candicans)

BALM OF GILEAD *(Populus candicans):* The closed buds of the poplar tree is the part used. It is an expectorant for chest ailments and bronchial disorders.

BASIL *(Ocimum basilicum):* The leaves are used. Basil aids in digestion and is used as a mild laxative. Since it also acts as a mild sedative, it is used to treat headaches.

KIDNEY BEANS *(Phaseolus vulgaris):* Tea made from the beans and pods are considered to be of diuretic nature. It helps to clean the kidneys and ureters of gravel.

BEE BALM *(Monarda didyma):* All of the plant can be used. Bee balm is used as an antiseptic because it contains thymol and removes impurities from the blood. Also used to stimulate the liver and spleen.

BLACKBERRY *(Rubus spp.):* Leaves, fruit, and roots are used for different illnesses. Dissolves deposits in the alimentary system as well as the kidneys.

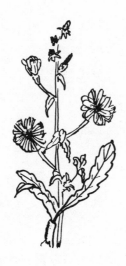

Chicory (Cichorium intybus)

BLUE COHOSH *(Caulophyllum thalictroides):* Anyone with high blood pressure should not take blue cohosh. It constricts the blood vessels of the heart. It does stimulate the uterus and is used extensively for female complaints.

BONESET *(Eupatorium perfoliatum):* The upper half of the herb is used. Has a cleansing effect upon all the organs. Used as a tonic as well as an aid in eliminating mucous from the alimentary, bronchial, bowel and liver systems. Also a muscle relaxant.

BORAGE *(Borago officinalis):* Leaves and flowers are used. Borage has a cucumber taste and makes a cooling addition to teas. Borage is often used to relieve depression. The flowers, made into a tea, are used to treat fevers and colds.

CALENDULA *(Calendula officinalis):* The flowers are used in remedies for many different illnesses. The tea is used internally and externally. It has been used to stop bleeding and has antibiotic properties to heal wounds. Use for chest ailments as well as for cramps, flu, stomach problems, and as an aid to induce sweating to bring down fever.

CATNIP *(Nepeta cataria):* Leaves and flowering tops are used to treat colic or flatulence.

CELERY *(Apium graveolens):* Tea made from celery eases the stomach and is used as a nervine and sedative. Always use fresh celery. Never use celery that is limp or discolored, even to cook with.

CHAMOMILE *(Matricaria chamomila):* The flowers and the upper half of the plant are used. It is a calmative and sedative. Treats headaches, cramps and other gastrointestinal disorders.

CHICORY *(Cichorium intybus):* The flowers are used as a sedative and general tonic. Also used as a diuretic.

CLEAVERS *(Galium aparine):* The entire herb is useful. A strong diuretic, it is used to dissolve deposits in the kidneys.

RED CLOVER *(Trifolium pratense):* The flowering tops are used. Great blood purifier and tonic. Most skin disorders are caused by impurities of the blood and this tea should be taken on a regular basis if you suffer from pimples, boils or other skin eruptions.

COLTSFOOT *(Tussilago farfara):* The leaves are the part used. This herb binds to toxins in the system and helps to eliminate them. Great expectorant.

COMFREY *(Symphytum officinale):* Roots and leaves are used. Great expectorant, demulcent, and emollient. Great tea for internal as well as external use.

CORN SILK: Corn silk is a great diuretic. Great to use to clean the urinary system and as a tonic for the whole system. Dry plenty of it so that you can use it during the winter months for kidney and bladder infections.

√ **DANDELION** *(Taraxacum officinale):* Roots and leaves are used. Use as a general tonic, as well as for liver and gallbladder complaints.

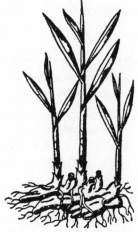

Ginger (Zingiber officinalis)

ELDER *(Sambucus canadensis):* Leaves, fruits and flowers are used. Elder flower tea is an excellent diuretic. Use for feverish colds, too.

SLIPPERY ELM *(Ulmus fulvus):* The dried inner bark is the part used. A mild expectorant, it soothes irritations of the alimentary and bronchial systems.

EYEBRIGHT *(Euphrasia officinalis):* Use the seeds as a help if you have a tendency toward kidney stones. Use in a rinse for eyes.

FENNEL *(Foeniculum vulgare):* All parts are used. Aids digestion and helps calm nervous stomach. Increases milk production.

FOXGLOVE *(Digitalis purpurea):* Originally this herb was used as a diuretic. Because kidney problems are closely allied with heart disease, the benefits to the heart was soon noticed. *Caution:* **I would not recommend that you use this to treat any illness.** Leave treatment of heart problems to your physician. It is mentioned here only for personal knowledge, not use.

FENUGREEK *(Trigonella foenum-graecum):* Use the seeds. Soothes the lining of the stomach and intestines.

WILD GINGER *(Asarum canadense):* The root is the part used. Wild ginger is a stimulant and diuretic. The herb acts on the kidneys to eliminate viscous matter. Also a great tonic for the whole body.

GINSENG: *(Panax quinquefolia):* The root is used. This is considered a near cure-all. Used as a tonic for all the systems of the body and has been used as an aphrodisiac for centuries.

GOLDENSEAL *(Hydrastis canadensis):* The root is used. Combined action on the stomach and liver.

HOREHOUND *(Marrubium vulgare):* The flowering tops and leaves are used. Use for bronchial and stomach disorders. Good for sore throats and colds. It is an expectorant.

HOLLYHOCK *(Althea rosea):* The roots and leaves are used. Leaves can be used uncooked in salads or cooked as a side dish. It is an emollient and good to use during colds. Use if prone to kidney stones.

IRISH MOSS *(Chondrus crispus,* and *gigartina mamillosa):* The dried plant is used. Use in bronchial disorders and for kidney problems. Use in cough syrups.

KELP *(Fucus vesiculosis):* Kelp contains iodine. Use to purify the blood as well as for goiters.

LAVENDER *(Lavandula angustifolia):* The flowers make a pleasant tea that has sedative properties. Use for releasing tension and headaches.

LEMON BALM *(Melissa officinalis):* The leaves make a tea with a sedative action. It is used to induce sweating to reduce fevers. It also regulates menstruation.

LEMON VERBENA *(Aloysia triphylla):* The leaves make a tea used for upset stomachs and has a tonic effect upon the intestines. It has a slight sedative effect and can be used to relax as well as reduce the fever of colds and flu.

PRICKLY LETTUCE *(Lactuca virosa,* and *L. scariola):* The leaves and gum are used. Use as a strong sedative to treat insomnia. Also removes hardened excretions from the bronchial system.

LICORICE *(Glycyrrhiza glabra):* The root is the part used. Has estrogen-like properties, so use during and after change of life. Use also for all blood and bronchial problems.

LOBELIA *(Lobelia inflata):* Use the herb after the seed capsule has opened. Used for asthma and bronchial disorders. *Caution:* As little as 50 mg of the dried herb has caused poisoning symptoms.

MARSH MALLOW *(Althaea officinalis):* The root is used to soothe inflammations and irritations of the urinary and alimentary systems. Will help to dispel hoarseness and tickling of the throat as well as help in all bronchial disorders.

MULLEIN *(Verbascum thapsus):* The flowers and leaves are the parts used most of the time. Every part can be used. Used for bronchial problems as well as to inhibit the growth of certain bacteria. It is great to use during colds, as it has antibiotic properties.

NETTLE *(Urtica dioica):* The leaves and upper part of the plant are used. Used to relieve arthritis pains. Also frequently used in remedies for losing weight.

NUTMEG *(Myristica fragrans):* Use in small doses to help stomach disorders and digestion. *Caution:* It is a powerful narcotic if used in too large a dose.

PANSY *(Viola tricolor):* The whole herb is used. A mild expectorant, used for colds and asthma. Good tonic for the heart. Pansy is also know as heartsease.

√ **PARSLEY** *(Petroselinum crispum):* The whole herb is used. Great diuretic. Parsley tea has long been used to treat kidney problems.

√ **PENNYROYAL** *(Hedeoma pulegioides):* The leaves of the herb are used in remedies. Relieves upset stomach and is a gentle stimulant. Good to use for menstrual cramps because it stimulates the uterine muscles.

PEPPERMINT *(Mentha piperita):* The leaves and the flowering tops
√ are the parts used. Removes hardened mucus from the alimentary and bronchial systems. Used for discomfort of colds and stomach problems.

PLANTAIN *(Plantago major):* The root and leaves are used. Plantain has antiseptic properties and removes toxins from the system.

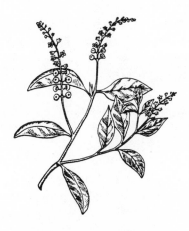

Pokeweed (Phytolacca americana)

POKEWEED *(Phytolacca americana):* The early shoots are used, as are the roots and berries. Pokeweed should be used with caution in any home remedy. I call it the chemotherapy of the herbs, as it is an extremely strong purge. It duplicates the effects of cortisone, which stimulates the entire glandular system. It is used only when drastic measures are called for and when all other natural methods have failed or are not suitable. It serves as a violent laxative and diuretic to clean the whole system. *Caution:* Please keep children away from the berries. It is not a safe plant for children to be around. They are fascinated by the beautiful berries.

PURSLANE *(Portulaca oleracea):* The herb above the ground is the part used. It is a good diuretic and cleanser for the kidneys. I have used it to give to goats that were suffering from scours (diarrhea). Make a tea with the purslane and then force it down their throats. It saved some of my goats from death.

RASPBERRY *(Rubus idaeus):* The leaves and fruit are used. Raspberry leaf tea stimulates the kidneys. The main purpose of the tea is to relax the uterine muscles, so it is considered a woman's herb. The roots are well known for their astringent properties. Because the root has concentrations of tannic and gallic acids, it has antibiotic value.

ROSE HIPS *(Rosa canina):* The hips, leaves and flowers are used. Great tonic for the blood. The hips contain vitamin P, which prevents and heals ruptures of small blood vessels. Treatment of the kidneys is indicated by the citric acids in the hips.

ROSEMARY *(Rosmarinus officinalis):* The needles are used as an astringent. It does relax the muscles and is used to treat depression, muscle spasms, and headaches.

SAGE *(Salvia officinalis):* Sage is a stimulating herb for the kidneys and helps to remove toxins from the system. The sedative properties are well known, so it can be used to treat headaches. Also used to treat colds because it removes catarrh in the alimentary and bronchial systems.

CLARY SAGE *(Salvia sclarea):* The leaves and seeds are used. Not only is clary sage used for eye disorders, but it has great properties that help to clear the sediments from the liver and kidneys. The tea is also used as a help for the stomach and intestines. Good for nausea and colic treatment.

SASSAFRAS *(Sassafras albidum)*: Bark of the root is most commonly used to break up the impurities in the blood system, so it is considered a blood purifier and thinner. It has a gentle, cleansing action that is helpful to the kidneys.

SKULLCAP *(Scutellaria laterifolia)*: The part above ground is used. The sedative properties are well known. Used for insomnia, nervous disorders and headaches.

SHEEP SORREL *(Rumex acetosella)*: The plant above-ground is used. Great to reduce fevers. It is used for blood disorders and cleans the urinary system. The word "sorrel" means sour. It is called sorrel for the acidity in the leaves.

SHEPHERD'S PURSE *(Capsella bursa-pastoris)*: The entire plant is used. It has a stimulating effect upon the uterine muscles. Also used in cases of diarrhea for humans and animals because of the astringent properties. It has hemostatic properties (stops bleeding), so it is useful for all kinds of hemorrhages affecting the uterine, lungs, stomach and kidneys. Shepherd's purse also increases the flow of urine and is helpful in removing mucous matter from the urine.

SOLOMON'S SEAL *(Polygonatum officinale)*: The root is the part used as a diuretic and it also has mucilaginous properties that help when vigorous expectoration is expected during bronchial disorders.

SPEARMINT *(Mentha spicata)*: Leaves and flowering tops are used. Great for treating colic and disturbances of the alimentary system. Used as a diuretic, also.

WILD STRAWBERRY *(Fragaria virginiana)* and **GARDEN STRAW-BERRY** *(Fragaria vesca)*: The root, leaves and berries are used. Drinking a tea made from strawberry leaves is a quick way to add minerals to the blood system. There is iron, potassium, sulfur, calcium, sodium and the associated acids, such as citric and malic, in the herb. The fruit contains vitamin C, so it is useful to treat scurvy. It is used to treat gout and related disorders. Has great benefits for the alimentary and urinary system. An all around fantastic tonic.

SWEET WOODRUFF: *(Galium odoratum):* The top part of the herb is used. Sweet woodruff has a very pleasant smell after it has started to dry. It has been used as a blood purifier, and as a tonic for the heart and the liver. It is also used as a calmative, helping to soothe stomach disorders and upsets.

GARDEN THYME *(Thymus vulgaris):* The whole top of the growing herb is used. Has a therapeutic action on the bronchial system. It is a stimulant and has antiseptic properties for use in cleaning the alimentary, urinary and bronchial systems.

VALERIAN *(Valeriana officinalis):* The root is the part used. Valerian has a very unpleasant smell, but it's influence on the brain and spinal cord are well-known. It acts like Valium without the side-effects of addiction that you would have with the prescription drug. It is a great calmative and is used extensively for sleeplessness and nervous disorders.

BLUE VERVAIN *(Verbena hastata):* The entire herb is used. The plant has diaphoretic and expectorant properties, so is great to use for chest complaints like pleurisy or for feverish colds.

VIOLET *(Viola odorata):* The flower, leaves and the roots are used. Violets contain more vitamin A than any other known plant. It's a great tonic and is a mild sedative,too. The roots of violets are known to soothe stomach pains and stop diarrhea.

WATERCRESS *(Nasturtium officinale):* The entire plant is used. Cleans the kidneys and is loaded with vitamin C. Contains many important minerals such as calcium, sulfur, copper, iron, and manganese, which strengthen the blood. Great tea to treat anemic conditions as well as being a great all around tonic.

WILLOW *(Salix spp.):* Contains salicin and salicylates that was the source of the first aspirin. Good to take for headaches, aches and pains of arthritic conditions, and relief of pain during menstruation. Good to use alone or mixed with other herbs to relieve discomfort of colds and flu.

WOAD *(Genista tinctoria)* The entire plant has a use. Not only does it supply us with the only natural blue dye (through use of the root), but the leaves supply us with a remedy for treating obstruction in the gall bladder and liver.

WILD YAM *(Dioscorea villosa):* Wild yam is treated by the body as though it is estrogen and so is of great help during menopausal stages. Used in the treatment of asthma and other ailments affecting the bronchial system.

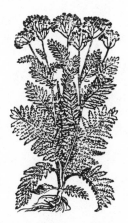

Yarrow (Achillea milefolium)

YARROW *(Achillea millefolium):* The whole herb is used. Great to use for feverish ailments. Contains silicin and salicylates, so it eases feverish aches and pains. Combine with other, more pleasant tasting herbs to make a tea. The roots are used to treat blood disorders. Yarrow has many minerals in it such as iron, calcium, potassium, sodium, and sulfur. It also contains two substances called achillein and achilleic acid. When ingested, these substances help to reduce the time that it takes for blood to clot. It has external uses as well. It is an astringent and can be used to clean—as well as relieve the pain of—wounds and sores.

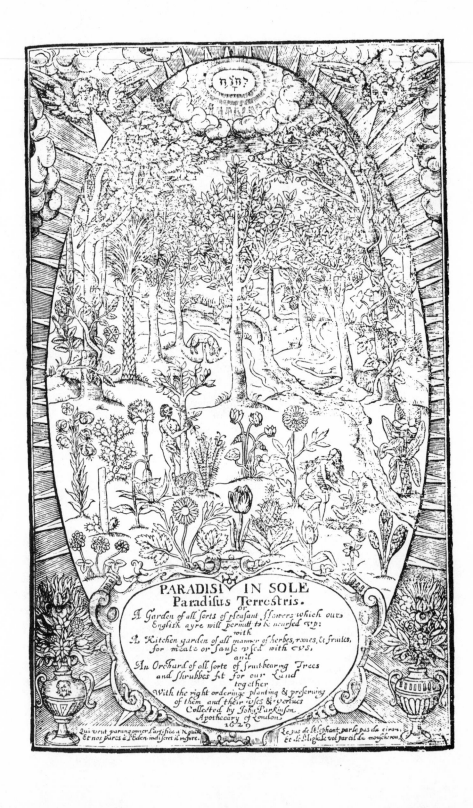

יהוה

PARADISI IN SOLE
Paradisus Terrestris.
Or
A Garden of all sorts of pleasant flowers which our
English ayre will permitt to be noursed vp:
with
A Kitchen garden of all manner of herbes, rootes, & fruites,
for meate or sause vsed with vs,
and
An Orchard of all sorte of fruitbearing Trees
and shrubbes fit for our Land
together
With the right orderinge planting & preseruing
of them and their vses & vertues
Collected by John Parkinson
Apothecary of London
1629

Qui veut parangonner l'artifice a Nature
Et nos parcs à l'Eden indiscret il mesure.

Le pas de l'éléphant par le pas du ciron,
Et le l'aigle le vol par celuy du mouscheron.

·6·

Tonics and Digestion

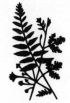

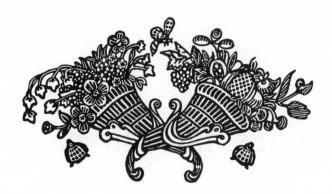

When we become aware of how much we are responsible for our own health, we soon realize that we are responsible for most of the illnesses that we contract. Health is very definitely a positive force and disease is exactly what it says, dis- ease of the body.

In many cases, illness is caused by a faulty diet. We all need tonics to keep the body supplied with certain minerals and vitamins in order to keep our immune system strong and healthy. If the immune system is in good order, then it is able to fight off certain illnesses with which we all come into contact. Then, if we do pick up a bug, our bodies can respond to the invading organisms much faster and we are able to start the healing process much more quickly. We may not be able to avoid an illness, but we can influence the length and severity of it. And we can stop the secondary infections that are sometimes part of a specific disease.

However, we do inherit susceptibilities to certain diseases. As we become more aware of just what our individual weaknesses are, we can begin to treat the body in such a way as to preserve its health. If there is a weakness in the respiratory system, then we know we have to work in order to keep that part as strong as possible. Because none of the body systems work alone, we must keep all the systems strong, simply because they do work with each other. Just think of your body as being a finely-tuned machine. If one part breaks down, the whole machine either breaks down completely or does not work to peak capacity. Life is to be lived to capacity, so the body has to be strong in order to fully enjoy all there is for us to be, do or have.

Herbs help strengthen the body so it can heal itself faster and in a more natural, healthy way. If you keep your body as free of chemicals as possible, the herbs have a better chance of getting right to the root of the problem. They can help the body to start working more efficiently in healing that specific disease.

Herbs are not a miraculously fast cure. Many times it does take a little longer for a specific herb to start working because herbs work at treating the underlying causes of the illness and because they do not work on just one specific symptom. It takes more time to balance several different systems. The herbs help the immune system to get a good balance so that the body is able to help in the healing process.

Tonics do take time to work on the system, so you want to continue the treatment for some time, to give the body time to adjust. We spend years neglecting the body and than are surprised when it fails to respond as fast as we think it should. It really does take more time for the body to heal than the length of an illness. You can begin to use tonics as a way to prevent illnesses instead of just treating a disease after the fact. Most of the tonics are stimulating, so if someone has been very ill, it is not a good idea to give tonics that are strong stimulants.

Using herbs to tone up your body is just one of the ways you can take responsibility for keeping the body in good working condition. I feel that it is one of the most important things you can do for yourself. The herbs tone up the organs that are affected by our digestive system. This helps your body to use all the natural vitamins and minerals that you get when you are careful to provide it with natural products and foods.

Just as the herbs can help us be balanced internally, we must look at ways we can be balanced externally, in our daily lives. All the money in the world cannot take the place of your health, and this is where balance in your lifestyle comes into play. I'm sure you have heard it said that all work and no play makes Jack a dull boy. Well, all play and no work can do the same thing. There should be time in your life for everything: work, play, quiet time, pleasure, people, love and many other joys. Be not a slave to any one activity and you will have some measure of control over your life. Learn to stop and smell the roses. Even though that is old advice, it is still good advice.

No one else is as vitally interested in preserving our health and the health of our families as we are. We know how we want our foods, and what we want in our foods better than anyone. When we preserve or prepare our own foods, we can take precautions to insure that the foods and herbs are handled properly and in a hygienic manner. We can make sure that what we ingest is as natural as possible.

What could be more natural than adding tonics to our daily life? Tonics are good to take all year. They can become part of your health-protecting diet. And they can really pick you up when you are feeling sluggish.

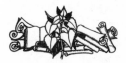

DANDELION TONIC: This is a good tonic for early spring. Pour 1 pint of boiling water over 1 ounce of dandelion flowers. Let steep covered for 10 minutes. Strain and sweeten. Drink several glasses a day for several days, or for as many days as you can before the flowers are gone.

The flowers also make a delicious jelly. The jelly tastes like honey and makes a really nice treat during the winter months. Why go to the trouble of getting rid of the dandelions when they are so useful in treating your body? They provide you with more than one food. The greens can be eaten and are quite delicious. They are full of vitamins and minerals that you can get in this natural way, instead of in pill form. The roots are also used as a tonic and make a good substitute for coffee.

FEVERFEW TONIC: Pour 1 pint boiling water over 1 ounce dried feverfew. Let steep 15 minutes, covered. Strain and sweeten. Drink in 1/2 cup doses for 1 day. This is a stimulant for the nervous system.

TONIC MIX: Mix together 1 ounce each of horehound, hyssop, licorice root, and marsh mallow root. Add 2 pints of water. Simmer until the liquid is reduced by 1/4. You should have about 1-1/2 pints of the tonic. Strain and dose with 1/2 cup of the liquid every couple of hours for 1 day of every week for a month. This tones up the respiratory tract and also stimulates and nourishes the adrenal glands.

SPRING TONIC: Pour 4 cups boiling water over 2 tablespoons of marjoram. Let it sit, covered for 15 minutes. Strain and sweeten. Up to two cups per day may be taken. *Caution:* This is a strong stimulant and should not be taken over once a day.

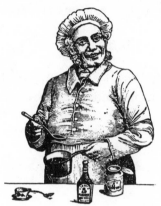

BLOOD-STRENGTHENING SPRING TONIC: Pour 1 quart of boiling water over 1 ounce each of burdock root, dandelion root, boneset herb, and sarsaparillas and boil for 15 minutes. Strain and drink 1 wineglass full 3 times a day. Continue treatment for 2-3 days. Refrigerate and drink cold. This is a great blood strengthener and purifier. It will also thin the blood while adding the extra, needed minerals.

TONIC FOR WOMEN: Mix 1/2 ounce each of strawberry leaves, plantain leaves, raspberry leaves and comfrey leaves. Add ginger if desired. Mix well and pour 1 cup boiling water over 1 teaspoon of the herb mixture. Strain and sweeten if desired. Drink several times daily for about a week.

No organ acts independently from other organs. This helps to tone up the reproductive organs and increases the health of tissues that relate to total health.

TONIC FOR MEN: Mix 1/2 ounce each of ginseng, shepherd's purse, corn silk and parsley. Mix well and add 1 teaspoon of the mixture to 1 cup of boiling water. Let steep 15 minutes, covered. Strain and sweeten if desired. Drink several cups per day for 1 week. This helps to tone up the male reproductive organs. The stimulation to the prostate is helpful to all parts of the system.

CHANGE OF LIFE TONIC: Mix 1 tablespoon each of hops, skull-cap, motherwort, chamomile, and gentian. Steep 1 teaspoon of the mix in 1 cup of boiling water for 15 minutes. Strain and sweeten. Drink several times daily. This tonic can be taken for symptoms as needed. Nervous irritation is one of the symptoms of menopause and this tea can be used to bring calmness to an agitated state.

ALL AROUND TONIC: This is a great tonic for the whole family. Simmer the peel of 3 lemons and 2 oranges in two quarts of water for 15 minutes, covered. Remove from heat and add 6 tablespoons of hops and 6 tablespoons of violet leaves and flowers. Steep for another 15 minutes. Strain and add honey to sweeten. Cloves may be added if desired. This tea has many vitamins, so it can be used as often as desired.

STIMULATE APPETITE: Pour 1 cup boiling water over 1 teaspoon tarragon leaves. Steep, covered, 10 minutes. Strain and sweeten with honey. Drink 1/2 hour before meals. Will also relieve flatulence if drunk after or during meals. Gas can be very uncomfortable and this does help to prevent buildup of gas in the intestines, as well as stimulating a poor appetite.

GENERAL TONIC: To build up your whole system, pour 1 cup of boiling water over 3 pumpkin blossoms and allow to steep, covered, 10 minutes. Strain and sweeten. This can be taken as often as desired as it provides many vitamins and minerals. Men can drink this tea as a tonic for the prostate gland.

VIOLET TONIC: This is a particularly good tonic for older folks and children. Violet leaves and flowers hold more vitamin A than any other leafy green. Add the chopped leaves and flowers to your salads. Make a tea using several teaspoons of the leaves and flowers to 1 cup of boiling water. Steep, covered, for 10 minutes. Strain, sweeten and drink as often as desired.

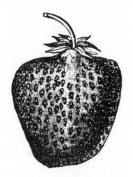

Strawberry (Fragaria vesca)

ALL AROUND TONIC: Wild strawberry leaves are chockful of vitamins and make a very good tonic. Dry the leaves for year round use. Pour 1 cup boiling water over 1 teaspoon of the dried leaves. Steep covered 10-15 minutes. Strain and sweeten. Drink several cups per day for 1 week if used as a tonic. Otherwise drink for enjoyment anytime.

WINE TONIC: Put 1 cup of sage in the blender and add 1 pint of burgundy or claret. Blend until sage is in very small pieces. Allow to age for several weeks and strain. Take during times of stress or as a general tonic by the tablespoon as needed.

SASSAFRAS SPRING TONIC: This is a good tonic to use in the spring as it thins out the blood as well as adding needed minerals. Everyone knows that sassafras has been used for centuries as a spring tonic. Try it, it's delicious.

To make the tea, add several teaspoons of sassafras root or bark to about 2 cups of boiling water. Allow to steep 15 minutes. Strain and sweeten. Drink several cups per day for 1 week. A commercial liquid of sassafras is available with certain substances removed. This you can make by following instructions on the bottle.

COMFREY TONIC AND FAST PICK-ME-UP: Put 2 leaves of comfrey in the blender along with 1 can frozen orange juice, adding water according to instructions on the can. Blend thoroughly. Very cooling and refreshing and very high in vitamins. Use only the tender new leaves for the full effect. This is great to use in the spring as a general tonic, and a refreshing cooling drink for the warmer months.

ALOE VERA TONIC: Many people place the juice from aloe vera in water and place in the refrigerator. Drink this as often as desired. Used as a general tonic and is a great bowel regulator.

ANOTHER GREAT TONIC AND BOWEL REGULATOR: A glass of cranberry juice is one of the best tonics I know. It can be used to clear up kidney and bladder infections and helps to regulate the bowels. It cleans the blood and helps the body to get rid of accumulated toxins. This helps to clear the complexion. Very high in potassium, which is needed by the body to dispose of waste materials and help keep the heart healthy. Cranberry juice is a good habit to get into. Drink in the morning with your breakfast meal.

BLOOD PURIFIER: Lightly steam chickweed and eat as a spinach substitute. Cleans impurities from the blood and acts as a tonic for the whole system.

INTERNAL CLEANSER: This is of special benefit to the blood and digestive system. Put nasturtium flower and leaves in salads. To make a good tonic tea, add a small handful of the flowers and leaves to 1 pint of boiling water and allow to steep for 30 minutes. Strain and drink several cups a day for 1 week to use as a tonic. Makes a nice peppery tea to drink just for the pleasure of the taste. Nasturtiums are a stimulant and a tonic. When the ripe buds of nasturtiums are dried and made into an infusion, they make a laxative that is fairly strong.

THIS IS A GREAT PURIFIER: Add 2 teaspoons watercress leaves to 1 cup of boiling water. Let steep 10-15 minutes. Strain and sweeten. Drink several cups per day for about a week.

BLOOD PURIFIER: Pour 1 pint of boiling water over a large handful of sheep sorrel leaves. Let steep 15 minutes. Strain and sweeten. Take for 1 week. This serves to internally cleanse the urinary system. It has been used for centuries to treat skin problems and eruptions. Also alleviates fevers and inflammatory disorders.

A GOOD STIMULANT: Add 3 tablespoons of angelica to 1 cup of boiling water. Cover and steep 10 minutes. This really perks you up. Take when you feel the need to add "get up and go" to your system. Aids in loosening and eliminating the catarrhal discharges from the urinary and bronchial systems. Good expectorant to use during colds and to treat chest complaints. Aids in eliminating gas, so would be used to treat colic and indigestion also.

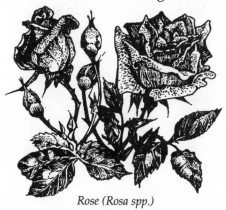

Rose (Rosa spp.)

ROSE HIP TONIC: Chop 2 teaspoons of rose hips and add to 2 cups of boiling water. Steep, covered, 15 minutes. Strain and sweeten. Can be used as is or added to other teas and fruit juices. Good to use if you have a cold as it adds extra vitamin C to your diet and will shorten the time of your illness.

COSTMARY TONIC: Costmary is also called Bible leaf. Add raw to salads or use to make an infusion of tea. Add a small handful of chopped leaves to 1 pint of boiling water. Steep 15 minutes, strain and sweeten. Excellent tonic for the liver. Take for 1 week if used as a tonic, drinking several cups per day.

TONIC TO STRENGTHEN THE LIVER AND SPLEEN: Simmer 1-1/2 cups of honeysuckle leaves and 1/2 cup of honeysuckle blossoms in 2 pints of water for 10 minutes. Strain and drink 2 cups a day before meals for 1 week. This is also good to use to help get rid of mucus during a cold.

SLUGGISH LIVER: To clean and stimulate the liver, drink 1 cup of beet juice daily for 1 week. I can my beets so that I have the juice handy year round.

LIVER TONIC: Mix together 1 ounce of chopped dandelion root with 1 ounce each of cinnamon bark, senna leaves, caraway seeds and ginger root. Add to 3 pints of water. Gently boil until liquid is reduced in volume to about 1-1/2 pints. Add 1/2 pound of sugar and return to boil. When it reaches the second boil, boil 2 minutes, remove from heat, strain, and cool. Store in the refrigerator. Dose frequently with 1 teaspoon daily for 1 week.

LIVER TONIC: Take a small handful of fresh watercress and pour 1 pint of boiling water over the herb. Cover and steep for 15 minutes. Strain and sweeten. A dash of fresh ginger can be added if desired. Drink warm several times daily for 1 week, if used as a liver tonic. Watercress is an astringent and stimulant, so it acts as a tonic for the urinary and alimentary systems.

BORAGE TONIC: Borage has been found to stimulate the adrenal glands. Adrenalin is released in the blood stream and this gives you extra energy. Put 1 tablespoon each of the flowers and chopped leaves of borage in 2 cups of boiling water. Steep 10 minutes, then strain and sweeten with honey. Take several cups daily for 1 week.

CARDIAC TONIC: Mix 1 tablespoon calendula, 2 tablespoons motherwort, 1 tablespoon cayenne, 1 tablespoon goldenseal and 4 tablespoons of hawthorn berries. Add 1 teaspoon of the herb mixture to 1 cup of boiling water. Cover and allow to steep 10 minutes. Strain and sweeten with honey. Drink several times daily for 1 week.

EDEMA: Edema is a swelling of the body tissues and results in excessive amounts of tissue fluid. It is sometimes called dropsy. There are many different areas of the body that edema may affect.

Diuretics are generally the accepted treatment as the fluid needs to be drawn from the body. Restricting salt intake is recommended, along with bed rest. The patient is placed on a diet that is rich in vitamins, low in salt and high in calories. Once large amounts of urine have been passed, the patient is placed on a regular diet.

Here is an old Irish remedy for dropsy that has been in use for centuries. Clean 2 potatoes thoroughly and peel. Add the peelings to 2 cups of water and bring to a boil. Reduce heat and simmer 15 minutes, covered. Strain and add 3 tablespoons of the liquid to a glass of water or cranberry juice. Drink 4 glasses daily until swelling has gone down.

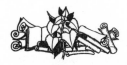

It sometimes helps to thin the blood, especially if you have heart problems. (*Caution:* If you are on heart medication, consult your doctor.) These are natural treatments to thin the blood. Vitamin C thins the blood. I believe it really wouldn't hurt to start taking it on a regular basis.

BLOOD THINNER: Ginger does as well to thin the blood as aspirin. It also reduces the pain for certain types of arthritis. It seems to help with rheumatoid arthritis especially well. Take 2 capsules every day. The empty capsules can be bought at a health food store or ordered through a company that handles herbs and health products. You can fill them yourself with powdered ginger.

HEART TONIC: Put 1 cup of grated honeysuckle root in 7 cups of water. Simmer gently 30 minutes. Strain, bottle, and refrigerate. Drink 2 cups daily for 1 week.

HEART TONIC: Pour 2 cups boiling water over 3 tablespoons of hawthorn berries. Steep overnight, covered. The next morning strain it, making sure to squeeze the berries to extract all the juice. Drink 1 cup, 2 times a day. Fresh or dried berries may be used. Take as long as desired, as a tonic.

FORTIFY HEART AND BRAIN: Place a small handful of fresh, wild rose petals or 3 tablespoons of dried rose petals in 2 cups of boiling water. Steep, covered, 15 minutes. Strain and sweeten with honey. Garden roses can be used if you have no access to the wild variety. Try to use the white roses from the garden if possible. Can be taken daily if desired.

STRENGTHEN HEART: Anyone with heart problems should eat all the honey they can. Put 1 tablespoon of chopped ginseng and 1 tablespoon of cinnamon in 1 pint of honey. Simmer 30 minutes. Strain and take by the tablespoon several times daily. Will increase blood circulation.

STRENGTHEN HEART: Violets are used to treat angina pectoris in Switzerland. Macerate 2 teaspoons of the leaves and add to 1 cup of boiling water. Steep covered 10 minutes. Strain and sweeten with honey. Take as often as desired.

STRENGTHEN HEART: Put 2 teaspoons of crushed rose hips in 1 cup of water. Bring to a boil and reduce heat. Gently boil for 3 minutes. Strain and sweeten with honey. Drink several times daily. Use this remedy as often as desired.

AIDS CONCENTRATION: Mix 3 tablespoons sage, 2 tablespoons goldenseal, 1 tablespoon cayenne, 8 tablespoons rosemary, 5 tablespoons yerba mate and 3 tablespoons skullcap. Add 1 teaspoon of the herb mix to 1 cup of boiling water and steep, covered, 10 minutes. Strain and sweeten. Drink twice daily for 2 weeks. Reduce to 1 cup daily. *Caution:* Some people show an allergic reaction to sage. Leave that out if desired.

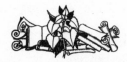

We all suffer from occasional indigestion and stomach upsets. Try some of these recipes until you find the one that works for you.

COLIC: Some babies seem prone to infantile colic in the first few months. It is caused by a spasm in any number of the soft organs and is accompanied by pain that can be quite severe at times. The infant will cry very loudly and draw the feet in toward the stomach. After giving an herb bottle, try letting the child lay stomach down on your lap. This seems to ease them. Many of the seed herbs help to bring relief. The infant normally grows out of the tendency so just hang in there and comfort the little person as best as possible.

COLIC TREATMENT: Mix 2 tablespoons each of the following: dill seed, fennel seed and anise seed. Add 2 tablespoons each of catnip and chamomile as a relaxant. Add 1 teaspoon of the mixture to 1 cup of boiling water. Let steep, covered, for 15 minutes. Strain well and dilute with same amount of water. Give to the child between feedings from a bottle.

COLIC: Steep 1 teaspoon each of chamomile herb and fennel seed in 1 cup of boiling water for 15 minutes, covered. Strain well and add 1/2 tablespoon of the liquid to the babies formula. Can be repeated up to 3 times a day if necessary.

VOMITING IN CHILDREN AND ADULTS: Toast 5 tablespoons of oatmeal under the broiler. Pour 1 pint of boiling water over the oats to make a thin gruel, adding sugar and cinnamon to sweeten. Drink as much as desired (and as often as needed) until vomiting is stopped. Will settle the stomach quickly.

NAUSEA: Pour 1 cup boiling water over 1 teaspoon dried chamomile and steep 10 minutes. Strain. Add 1/4 teaspoon cinnamon to the tea before adding sugar to taste.

STOMACH CRAMPS: Lemon balm tea is used to help with cramps. Put 6-8 lemon balm leaves in 1 cup of boiling water. Steep covered for 10 minutes and strain. Sweeten and drink warm. Ginger may be added for extra help, if desired.

DIGESTIVE AID: Place 1/2 ounce of powdered sea kelp in 2 cups of boiling water and allow to steep for 15 minutes. Drink as needed for indigestion.

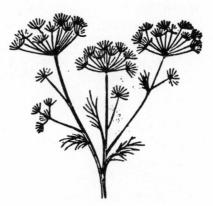

Dill (Anethum graveolens)

DILL SEED TEA: This one is good for indigestion. Bruise 2 teaspoons dill seeds and leaves. Cover with 1/2 pint boiling water. Let steep, covered, until cool. Strain and sweeten. Take about 2 ounces every hour until indigestion is alleviated.

NERVOUS INDIGESTION: Pour 1 cup of boiling water over several sprigs of marjoram and allow to steep, covered, 10 minutes. Strain and sweeten with honey. Also good for headaches brought on by nervous tension.

INDIGESTION AID: Pour 1 cup of boiling water over 1 teaspoon of hop flowers and add 1 tablespoon of glycerin. Steep for 5 minutes. Strain and drink 30 minutes before your meal. Sweeten as desired.

COFFEE HELPER: Coffee can be good to aid indigestion after a meal. It can also curb the appetite if you drink a cup 1/2 hour before meals.

PARSLEY TEA: Make a tea using 2 cups of fresh parsley to 1 quart boiling water. Let sit, covered, until cool. Strain and reheat as needed. Sweeten to taste. This is good to help settle the stomach, as well as being a great diuretic for the kidneys.

BINGO MIX: Mix together 1 tablespoon each of fennel seed, aniseed, coriander seed and caraway seed. Bruise 1 teaspoon of this mixture. Pour 1/2 pint of boiling water over the bruised seed, cover and allow to steep until cool. Sweeten and drink warm or cool. Settles indigestion fast.

MARSH MALLOW TEA: Pour 1 pint of boiling water over 1 ounce of dried marsh mallow leaves. Steep, covered, until cool. Strain and flavor with ginger if desired. Reheat as needed. Great for indigestion.

THIS ONE IS ESPECIALLY GOOD AFTER MEALS: Mix together 1 cup each of fennel seed, dill seed and leaves, chamomile flowers, aniseed and spearmint leaves. Pour 1 cup of boiling water over 1 teaspoon of the herb mixture. Cover and steep 10 minutes. Strain and sweeten. Drink warm after all meals to aid indigestion.

BALM FOR UPSET STOMACH: Pour 1 cup of boiling water over 1 teaspoon lemon balm. Steep for 15 minutes, covered. Strain and sweeten. Lemon balm has a very calming and soothing effect. Good tea to use during pregnancy, when you feel nauseous. Also a good tea to use before going to bed as it helps to relax you.

DIGESTION HELP: Drinking papaya juice seems to relieve digestion problems. Drink after meals to prevent upsets.

DIGESTIVE PROBLEMS: Sprinkling cayenne pepper liberally over your food will help tremendously in all digestive problems. Continue the treatment until the problem is solved. Cayenne can also be used as a tea or in #00 capsules to solve digestive problems. Simply add 1/2 teaspoon of cayenne pepper to 1 cup of hot water. Drink several cups a day. You wouldn't think that using cayenne pepper would help ease a stomach disorder, but it really does help.

SETTLES UPSET STOMACH: Mix together 1 teaspoon goldenseal, 1 heaping teaspoon chamomile, 1 teaspoon mullein, 1 teaspoon skullcap, 2 teaspoons lobelia, 1 tablespoon mint, 1/4 tea-spoon powdered peppermint, and 1 tablespoon pennyroyal. Add 1 teaspoon of this herbal mixture to 1 cup of boiling water and allow to steep 10 minutes. Strain and sweeten. Settles stomach quickly.

FLATULENCE: Drink this tea cold. Pour 1 quart of boiling water over 2 ounces of honey and 1 ounce of bruised sage leaves. Steep covered several hours or at least until the liquid is cool. Strain and refrigerate. Use this as often as needed to relieve gas.

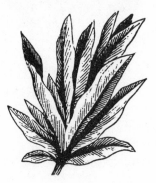

Sage (Salvia officinalis)

FLATULENCE: Peppermint tea is good tasting and good for your digestive system. Drink after meals to help ease digestive upsets and prevent gas buildup. Put 1 teaspoon of peppermint leaves in 1 cup of boiling water. Steep covered 15 minutes and strain. Sweeten as desired. Drink hot or cold.

LEMON HEARTBURN TREATMENT: Try adding 2 teaspoons of lemon juice in 1/2 cup of warm water. Sip to relieve heartburn.

HEARTBURN: Pour 1 cup of boiling water over 1 teaspoon of dried peppermint leaves. Let steep, covered, 10 minutes. Sweeten with honey after straining. Drink warm, reheating as necessary to relieve heartburn.

HEARTBURN TREATMENT: This is an unusual treatment, but I've had several people to report that it does work. Take 1 table-spoon of brown sugar to relieve the pain of heartburn.

RELIEF FROM HEARTBURN: If you suffer from heartburn often, try eating a bowl of oatmeal on a daily basis. Stops heartburn from occurring.

HEARTBURN: Eating raw carrots or a stalk of celery after meals helps to stop heartburn.

TREATMENT OF STOMACH ULCERS: Red clover tea relieves pain from ulcers and mild indigestion. It helps to relieve excess acidity. Also used to treat rickets as it replaces essential minerals. Red clover has lots of calcium and phosphorus and this helps to strengthen teeth and bones. Drink 1 cup before meals and at bedtime. Add 2 tablespoons of dried or fresh red clover to 1 cup of boiling water and allow to steep, covered, 10 minutes. Strain and sweeten with honey.

STOMACH ULCER TREATMENT: Drink fresh goat's milk to prevent or treat ulcers. It's very good for you. Many people say that they won't drink goat milk because of the taste. The reason for the different taste is simple. One of the reasons has to do with the way that the milk is treated.

The milk should be strained and cooled immediately after you have milked. Cooling the milk as fast as possible is probably the main secret to avoiding the funny taste that so many people associate with goat's milk. It is really very tasty if processed properly.

Another reason for the funny taste could be the nanny's close proximity to a billy goat. Never keep your nannies in with or close to a billy. I never bothered to keep billies because I found it easier to have the nannies bred rather than having the hassle of keeping the little buggers.

When the time has come to breed your nanny goat, get a cloth and rub it all over a billy, so that his scent is transferred to the cloth. I keep the cloth in a tightly closed jar, to preserve its scent. I allow the nanny to smell the cloth to get a good indication of her readiness to accept a billy. Many times it seemed to put them in the mood. Anyway, back to the milk.

Many people who do not tolerate cow milk or who suffer from allergies do very well drinking goat milk. I first got interested in using goat milk when my granddaughter was born. She had an intolerance to cow's milk and she did not do very well on soy milk. We put her on the fresh goat milk and she did very well.

STOMACH ULCER TREATMENT: This is another good Irish treatment. After boiling potatoes, save the water and drink this. It will cure ulcers if done on a daily basis.

STOMACH ULCER TREATMENT: Mix 1 teaspoon of cayenne pepper with 1 cup of hot water. Drink up to 3 cups per day. Will stop the pain overnight. Continue until ulcers no longer bother you.

STOMACH ULCER TREATMENT: Eating yogurt on a daily basis will prevent or cure stomach ulcers, as it destroys harmful bacteria that causes the formation of acids in the stomach.

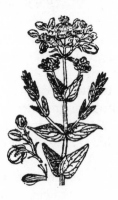

St. John's Wort (Hypericum perforatum)

GALL BLADDER TREATMENT: St. John's wort tea is good to use if you have gall bladder trouble. Make a tea using 4-5 leaves steeped in 1 cup of boiling water. Strain, and drink several times a day to soothe the gall bladder. *Caution:* St. John's wort can cause photosensitivity and the skin will be very sensitive to sunlight. Do not use if you already suffer from sensitivity to sunlight. If you are using it to treat gall bladder, please stay out of the sun during treatment. Do not use the treatment for long periods of time. Use only when you are having problems with your gall bladder.

GALL BLADDER TREATMENT: Gall bladder pain is reduced if you take 1 tablespoon of olive oil before each meal.

GALL BLADDER TONIC: Take 4 tablespoons of lemon juice every morning on an empty stomach. Continue for at least 1 week to get results.

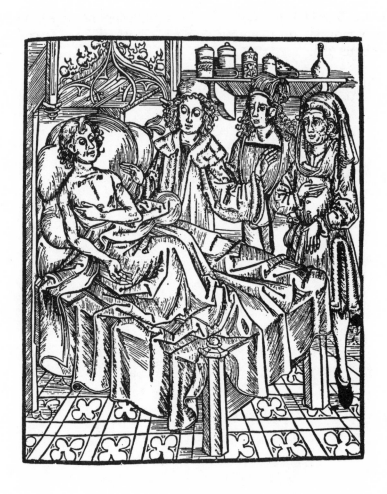

·7·

Ear, Eye, Nose and Throat Complaints

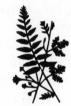

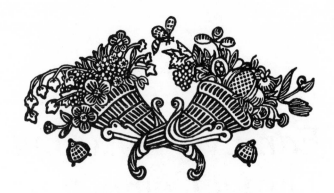

The things we hear, see, smell and taste make our lives interesting. So, whenever any of these senses is dulled or impaired by illness, it makes our world a little grayer. Luckily, Mother Nature provides us with different kinds of herbs to help remedy the situation. Over the years, we humans have managed to take nature's gifts and make them into good remedies.

EARACHE REMEDIES: Heat seems to help stop earache pain. Place a warm damp washcloth over the ear and lay ear on a heating pad to keep warm. Pain that persists should be seen by your physician, as it could signal an ear infection or eardrum perforation.

If an insect is lodged in the ear, do not attempt to remove the bug with any instrument or use a bright light to lure the insect out. This sometimes causes the insect to burrow deeper into the ear. You should fill the ear with a bland oil and float the insect out. If you are unsuccessful in this, you should go to your physician for help.

Sometimes water will become trapped in the ear after swimming. Tilting the head and then tapping it sharply will usually discharge the water. If not, then you may want to put several drops of 70% isopropyl alcohol in the ear. This helps to evaporate the water. Sometimes the feeling of water in the ear is caused by swelling of the cerumen. You should consult your physician for that problem.

KEEP THIS MIXTURE HANDY FOR EARACHES: Steep 1/4 cup of mullein flowers in 1/2 cup of olive oil for several weeks. Strain several times. Store tightly covered. When you are ready to use it, warm the oil. It should be about room temperature (don't use it cold). Make sure it is merely warm, *not hot*. Put several drops of the oil in the affected ear. Apply a warm cloth to ear. It wouldn't hurt to put sterile cotton plugs in the ear after putting in the drops.

EARACHE TREATMENT: Warm some olive or castor oil and put several drops of it in the affected ear. Place a piece of sterile cotton in the ear.

EARACHE: Mix 1 teaspoon each of witch hazel and glycerin. Warm the mixture and saturate a piece of cotton with it. Place in the ear and keep warm.

EARACHE: Warmed honey, applied a few drops at a time into the affected ear, will help to stop an earache. Place a cotton ball in the ear after applying the honey to keep in the warmth.

INNER EAR DISORDERS: Grind 1 teaspoon fresh ginger. Add 1 cup boiling water. Steep 15 minutes and strain. Sweeten with honey and drink as a tea. Controls motion sickness, nausea, and vertigo caused by inner ear disorder.

NAUSEA OR VERTIGO: Chewing fresh mint leaves relieves feelings of nausea.

MOTION SICKNESS: Sometimes chewing 4-5 whole cloves will relieve motion sickness.

EAR RINGING: Ear ringing or tinnitus has several causes. The most common is caused by the overuse of aspirin or other drugs. Many times it occurs in certain diseases of the exterior, middle or inner ear. Consult with your physician as he or she can ascertain what the source is, if you do not take any medication on a regular basis. While I have never tried it, it is said that putting a few drops of onion juice in the ear will stop earache and ear ringing.

TREATMENT FOR TINNITUS: Mix 1 tablespoon of turpentine and 1 tablespoon almond or olive oil. Saturate a cotton ball with the oil and place in the ear overnight.

TINNITUS: Put 6 large cloves of garlic in the blender, adding 1 cup of olive or almond oil. Blend until the garlic is minced. Put in a glass jar and allow to steep, covered, for 1 week. Strain and apply several drops in the ear to stop the ringing and aid in hearing.

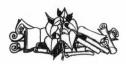

Eye care is important, so I've included a few recipes for eye washes. Any serious problems should be seen by your physician. Your eyesight is a very precious gift.

SAID TO IMPROVE SIGHT: Add a small handful of cornflower blossoms to 1 cup of boiling water. Allow to steep 30 minutes. Strain and use as an eye wash. Good tea to use for conjunctivitis. Conjunctivitis has many causes. Sometimes it is caused by allergies (if it happens in the spring). Certain types of conjunctivitis are caused by foreign matter in the eye. Several viral agents can also cause it. Pinkeye is highly contagious and is most often found in children, although adults can be affected also.

HELPS PREVENT CATARACTS: Mix 2 teaspoons each of honey and apple cider vinegar with a glass of water. Drink with every meal. Also said to retard cataract growth, as well as to prevent them.

CATARACTS: To help retard cataract growth, put a drop of honey in the corner of each eye on a nightly basis. May take several months before improvement is noticed.

POULTICE TO USE FOR BLACK EYES: Place a handful of chopped leaves and stems of hyssop in 2 cups of boiling water. Allow to steep for 30 minutes. Strain and dip clean cloth in herb liquid and apply to black eye.

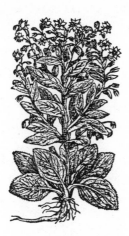

Borage (Borage officinalis)

EYE WASH: Borage eyewash can clear redness stemming from eye strain and fatigue. Use as a gentle wash. Pour 1 cup of boiling water over 1 teaspoon of dried borage leaves. Steep until cool. Strain and put in sterile jar. Use a few drops directly in the eye or use as a compress. Relieves puffiness around the eyes.

EYE WASH: Add 1 teaspoon of eyebright to 1 cup boiling water. Let steep 15 minutes. Strain well and cool. Use this as an eye wash. Fennel, elder flowers, or verbena can also be used. Helps tired eyes and eye strain. Very helpful when conjunctivitis is present.

EYE WASH: Mix 1 teaspoon of honey with 1/4 cup of hot water. Cool the mixture slightly and use with eye cup for gentle wash.

BLOODSHOT EYES: Apply a few drops of castor oil to the eyes to clear the redness from them.

INFLAMED EYES: Pour 1 cup boiling water over 2 tablespoons of yarrow flowers. Steep for 10 minutes. Strain and dip clean cloth in liquid and apply to eyes as a compress.

FRESHEN EYES THAT ARE IRRITATED BY STRAIN: Use 1/2 teaspoon calendula to each cup of boiling water. Let stand until cool. Strain well and put in sterile bottle. Dip a cotton ball in this liquid squeezing out excess liquid. Place over the eyes for 10-15 minutes as a compress.

EYE WASH: Add 1 teaspoon fennel seed to 1 cup boiling water. Let steep 15 minutes. Strain several times and use the liquid to rinse the eyes with an eye cup. With the leftover liquid, soak a clean cloth and use as a compress over the eye for 15 minutes.

EYE WASH: Add 1 teaspoon each of parsley and calendula to 2 cups of boiling water. Steep, covered, 10 minutes. Strain several times. Use in eye cup. Refrigerate for later use in tightly closed bottle. Warm as necessary. Do not use too hot or too cold.

EYE WASH: Put 1-1/2 teaspoons of baking soda in 3/4 cup of warm water. Use as an eye wash.

EYE WASH: Put 1 teaspoon of fennel, elder flowers, or verbena in 1 cup of boiling water. Cool, strain well, and use as an eye wash. Helps tired eyes and is helpful when conjunctivitis is present.

EYE CARE: Put 1/4 teaspoon each of fennel, eyebright and chamomile in 2 cups hot water. Let steep until cool. Strain through sterile cotton balls to catch any particles that might irritate the eye. Use as an eye wash for sore or inflamed eyes.

EYE IRRITATION: To obtain immediate relief from eye irritation, put 1 drop of castor oil in the eye. Relieves the pain fast.

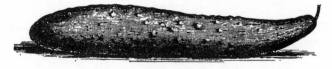

Cucumber

CUCUMBER TONIC FOR EYES: Slice a cucumber and place slices over the eyes. Leave on for 15 minutes. This refreshes and relieves puffiness around the eyes.

TONIC FOR EYES: Soak a cotton ball in witch hazel. Put the poultice over the eyes for 20 minutes. This relieves irritation caused by tired or strained eyes.

TREATMENT OF STIES: Sties are caused by bacterial infections. They cause a localized swelling of one of the sebaceous glands of the eyelid. The external sties are superficial and seem to be not too serious. The internal sties are a matter for your physician to treat. Applying hot packs frequently to the eye usually brings about drainage and resolution.
Put 1 teaspoon of tansy in 1 cup of boiling water. Steep 10 minutes and dip cloth in the herb liquid. Apply to the eye affected as a compress.

TREATMENT OF STIES: Steam fresh cabbage leaves until just limp. Drain and apply warm as a compress to the affected eye. Leave on for about 15 minutes, covered to keep warm. This is an old Irish treatment and seems to work.

TREATMENT OF STIES: Scrape a raw potato and place on the affected eye as a poultice. This is another Irish treatment. Amazing what the common potato can be used for, isn't it?

TREATMENT OF STIES: Moisten a pekoe tea bag with boiling water and apply to the affected eye as a poultice. Cover with a loose bandage and leave on for several hours. Repeat as necessary.

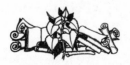

THROAT AND MOUTH COMPLAINTS: Often, the bleeding of the gums can signify scurvy or an inflammation, such as trench mouth. Here are some guidelines: Look at the bottom edge of the teeth, at the gum line, and notice the coloration. If there is a bluish-red tint, it would signify lead poisoning. A blue tint alone would indicate silver poisoning. A greenish line may indicate copper poisoning; a red line may signify gingivitis, pyorrhea, or scurvy. A purplish line does indicate scurvy. If the gum is spongy, you should see your physician immediately as it could indicate any number of diseases that would need his or her attention.

INFECTED GUMS: To treat infected or inflamed gums, take a mouthful of papaya juice and hold it in the mouth for 10 minutes. It heals the tissue of the gums.

An irritation of the gum can cause it to be red, swollen, and tender. This can be caused by dentures or injury to the mouth.

BLEEDING GUMS: Wet 1/2 teaspoon of myrrh to make a paste. Apply to gums before bed. You will notice quite an improvement in the morning.

MOUTH WASH FOR CANKER SORES: Canker sores (or "stomatitis" as they are sometimes called) have many causes. They may be caused by bacteria or viruses, irritants such as alcohol and tobacco, or by sensitization to chemical substances in toothpastes or commercial mouthwashes. They can also be caused by iron or vitamin deficiencies, especially from a lack of folic acid and vitamin B-12.

If canker sores occur in infants, the milk should be sterilized before giving it to the child and the mouth should be washed frequently, using a fresh cloth each time.

Adults should attempt to correct any disturbances of the gastric system. Also, using a weak solution of boric acid as a wash seems to help. If that is not available, use thyme, as it is a very good astringent. Pour 1 cup boiling water over 1 teaspoon thyme and steep covered 15 minutes. Strain and use as a gargle.

CANKER TREATMENT: Put 2 teaspoons of baking soda in 1 glass of water and use the solution to rinse the mouth and relieve the pain.

CANKER TREATMENT: Add 1 teaspoon of cinquefoil to 2 pints water. Boil gently until liquid is halved. Strain well, adding 2 tablespoons of borax to herb mixture. Use as a mouth wash. Do not swallow.

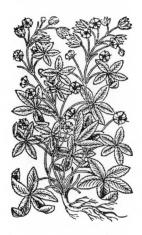

Cinguefoil (Potentilla reptans)

THRUSH TREATMENT: Thrush is caused by the growth of Candida albicans in the mouth or throat. It is characterized by the formation of white patches or sores. It is found most often in young children and can cause fever and pain. My father had the gift of being able to blow into the mouth of the person affected with thrush and it would go away. I recall several people throughout my life who had this gift. I don't try to explain how or why they were able to do so, just that it did work.

Apple cider vinegar also works as an astringent and can be used to cleanse the mouth. Rinse the mouth with half water and half apple cider vinegar every couple of hours to relieve pain and help heal.

THRUSH TREATMENT: Put yogurt in the mouth and hold it in as long as you can. Eating yogurt will help to prevent any gastric upset that will cause cold sores or thrush.

THRUSH TREATMENT: Put 1 tablespoon each of rosemary and sage in 1 cup of boiling water. Steep until cool. Strain and use as a mouth wash every 1/2 hour.

THRUSH TREATMENT: Put 1 tablespoon of dried mint and 2 teaspoons of thyme in 1 cup of boiling water. Steep 30 minutes. Use as a mouth wash.

TREATMENT FOR THRUSH: Pour 1 cup boiling water over 1/2 ounce red raspberry leaves. Cover and steep until cool. Strain well and apply to inside of mouth with a swab several times daily.

THRUSH TREATMENT: Rub the white patches with alum to help heal and relieve pain.

COLD SORE RELIEF: Add 2 teaspoons of red clover to 1 cup of boiling water. Allow to steep until cool. Strain and dip cloth in the tea. Apply to the cold sore repeatedly for 15 minutes several times a day.

COLD SORE TREATMENT: Apply buttermilk to the cold sore to help dry it up.

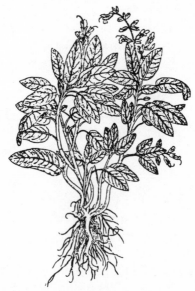

Sage (Salvia officinalis)

COLD SORE TREATMENT: Add 1 teaspoon of dried sage to 1 cup of boiling water. Allow to steep 15 minutes. Strain and add 1 teaspoon of ginger and honey to sweeten. Drink 3 cups throughout the day. Brings relief within 24 hours.

TOOTHACHES: Put several drops of vanilla directly on the affected tooth.

TOOTHACHE: Mix 1/2 teaspoon each of salt and alum. Pack in and around the tooth for quick pain relief.

TOOTHACHE: Soak a cotton ball with oil of cloves and apply on the tooth.

TOOTHACHE: Soak a cotton ball in ammonia and place over the affected tooth.

TOOTHACHE: Garlic is said to stop a toothache. Place a small piece of the garlic clove directly into the cavity of the tooth.

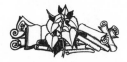

SINUS TREATMENT: Run water until very cold. Mix together 2 cups of cold water with 1 tablespoon of Epsom salts and 2 teaspoons of bicarbonate of soda. Dip clean cloth in the liquid and place over sinus area. Replace to keep area cold. Relieves stuffy nose fast. Good to use during a cold.

SINUS TREATMENT: Put 1 teaspoon of dried rose petals in 1 cup of boiling water. Steep until cool. Strain and dip cotton ball in the liquid. Apply to the eyes as a compress for 15 minutes. Place drops directly in the eyes with an eyedropper if desired. Relieves sore, irritated eyes caused by sinus problems very well.

SINUS TREATMENT: Chewing honeycaps from the combs of honey is said to cure sinus problems.

SINUS TREATMENT: Simmer 2 tablespoons of crushed fenugreek seeds in 2 cups of water for 30 minutes. Strain and add 1 tablespoon each of lemon and onion juice. Drink several cups a day.

SINUS PROBLEMS: Dissolve one 500 mg vitamin C tablet in 1/4 cup of warm water. Apply directly into the nostril with an eyedropper using 1/2 dropperful for each side, 2 times a day. My husband had a chronic infection of the sinus and we tried using this twice daily. I'm happy to say it works very well.

SINUS CONGESTION: Eat 2 garlic cloves 3 times a day for a week. Sinuses should start draining toward the end of the week.

BONESET FOR SINUS CONGESTION: This may take several days to loosen up congestion. Pour 1 cup boiling water over 1 teaspoon of boneset. Cover and steep 15 minutes. Strain and sweeten. Drink with every meal and before bed.

TO CLEAN SINUS PASSAGE DURING A COLD: Add 1 ounce mullein herb and 1 tablespoon of balm of Gilead to a kettle of boiling water. Inhale the steam.

TO CLEAR STUFFY NOSE: Place several trays of ice cubes in a basin of water and place only the toes in the water until numb. Sounds crazy, but it works.

STUFFY NOSE: Put 1/4 cup lemon thyme in 1 quart of water. Boil and inhale the steam. This clears a stuffy nose.

STUFFY NOSE: Add 1 ounce of chopped comfrey root (or the leaves if the root is unavailable) to 1 cup water. Bring to a boil and inhale the steam to relieve a stuffy nose. Cover the head and basin with a towel to get the full effect.

TO CLEAR HEAD COLDS: Mix 1/2 cup each of apple cider vinegar and water. Bring to a boil and inhale the fumes.

COLDS AND SORE THROATS: Sore throats are caused by an inflammation of the tonsils, larynx or pharynx. Keep the patient warm and comfortable and give plenty of fluids while treating sore throats and colds. A sore throat can be painful and uncomfortable, so be as understanding as possible to the patient. Many times my patience is tried sorely by my husband when he is ill. Men seem to take a simple illness much differently than women do. Bless their hearts, they deserve some waiting on when they are ill, but they also may exaggerate the symptoms in order to get more sympathy than warranted.

During the winter months, many people have sore throats, especially if there are young ones around that attend school. At the first sign of a sore throat, try gargling with peroxide and water. This generally stops a sore throat in it's track. For those sore throats you do not manage to catch early enough to nip them in the bud, try several of these recipes. Follow the old standby of rest, plenty of fluids and go on a light diet.

VINEGAR TREATMENT FOR COLDS AND SORE THROATS: Mix 2 cups vinegar with 1 cup of honey. Drink a wineglass of this mixture 3 times daily.

TREATMENT FOR SORE THROATS: Gargle with raw beet juice to relieve a sore throat.

ONE OF THE BEST I'VE FOUND FOR SORE THROATS: Make a paste using 1 tablespoon slippery elm powder, and just enough water to make a paste. Dissolve 1/2 cup of honey in 1 pint of boiling water. Add honey water slowly to slippery elm paste. Take 1 tablespoon as needed.

ALOE VERA GARGLE: Put several leaves of aloe vera in an enamel pan. Add several pints of water and bring to a boil. Strain well and use as a gargle.

RELIEVE SORE THROATS: Dry a pomegranate rind. Add 2 tablespoons of the dried and grated pomegranate rind to 2 cups of water. Bring to a boil and reduce heat. Simmer the mixture until halved. Strain and add 1/4 cup of sugar. Gargle with the liquid as needed.

BORAGE TEA FOR SORE THROATS: Make a tea using 1/2 cup of borage leaves to 1 pint of boiling water. Steep for 30 minutes. Strain and refrigerate. Use as a gargle when needed for sore throats.

SORE THROAT: Anise mint tea is very good for sore throats. Use 1 teaspoon dried anise mint for each cup of boiling water. Let steep 10 minutes. Strain and sweeten. Drink as warm as possible.Repeat as often as desired.

SORE THROAT TREATMENT: Add 1/2 cup of brown sugar to 1/2 cup of brandy. Mix well and sip as needed to relieve a sore throat.

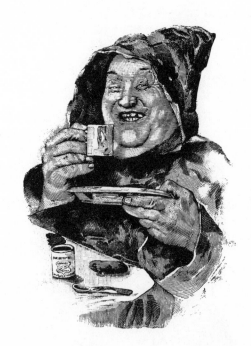

CAYENNE TREATMENT FOR COLDS AND SORE THROATS: Mix 1 teaspoon cayenne pepper with 1 cup boiling water. Drink 3

times daily to stop or ward off colds and sore throats. This really does work very well. The length of the illness is drastically reduced.

GARGLE FOR SORE THROATS: Use this at the first hint of a sore throat. Mix 2 tablespoons honey, 1/2 teaspoon cayenne pepper, 4 tablespoons apple cider vinegar, and 1 tablespoon of lemon juice to 1 cup warm water. Mix well and use as a gargle.

SWOLLEN GLANDS: Put 5 leaves of ivy in 1 cup of boiling water and simmer for 10 minutes. Strain and cool. Take 1 tablespoon 3 times a day.

INFLAMED OR INFECTED TONSILS: Place a large handful of sage in 1 pint of water. Simmer for 15 minutes or until sage is soft. Dip a flannel cloth in the liquid and place the sage leaves in the flannel before wrapping around the throat. Dip another cloth in the liquid, wrap this, too, around the throat. Keep replacing the outer cloth to keep the first poultice warm. Give a strong infusion of sage tea to drink during treatment. Swellings and inflammation should subside within hours.

SORE THROAT GARGLE: Place 2 tablespoons of chopped blackcurrant leaves in 1 cup of water. Simmer for 15 minutes. Strain and cool. Use as a gargle to relieve sore throat.

SORE THROAT GARGLE: Pour 1 pint of boiling water over 1 ounce of dried sage and 1/2 teaspoon of cayenne pepper. Steep overnight and use as a gargle.

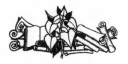

ALLERGIES: Many people suffer from allergies. An allergy is caused by an acquired hypersensitivity to a substance that would not ordinarily cause a reaction. There is often a genetic predisposition to acquire a particular allergy.

I had never suffered from allergies until a neighbor sprayed his field with an herbicide and I had the misfortune to be close to the area. The wind brought the spray over my way and enveloped me in a cloud, while covering my garden as well. I lost my supply of ladybugs that I had been so careful to build up over time. I also suffered from severe bronchial asthma for several years. The incident made me really aware of the way we treat our environment and the effects that it has on each and every one of us.

Some of the common allergic reactions may include eczema, bronchial asthma, hay fever, and food allergies. I believe the cases of asthma are more frequent now and more people are dying from it. I think this is linked to the amount of artificial chemicals with which we are surrounded.

We should all fight the use of the pesticides and herbicides a little harder. This junk is getting in our water supplies and will eventually affect all of us. The increase of asthma is just the first sign that something must be done now to control use and abuse of chemical substances. We must stop harming Mother Nature and stop passing these chemicals through the food chain to our children. We have to prevent our families from putting artificial chemicals in and on their bodies. Our exposure to the chemicals builds up and causes us to suffer hypersensitivity to substances. Control what goes on in your home first and you will soon want to have some say-so in what everyone else is doing to control your environment.

Here are some recipes to help you control allergies.

FOR CHEST CONGESTION AND WHEEZING CAUSED BY ALLERGIES: Take 500 mg of vitamin B-6 twice a day to bring relief. You should get improvement within a month. It would help to take 500 mg of vitamin C daily while on this treatment.

HONEY AND VINEGAR TREATMENT: Mix 2 tablespoons each of honey and vinegar with a glass of water. Drinking this mixture with every meal will help relieve symptoms.

BEE POLLEN TREATMENT: Bee pollen strengthens the respiratory system and is good to treat allergies. Take 1 teaspoon of granules or the equal of 4 capsules every day.

·8·

Headaches and Sedatives

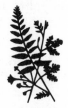

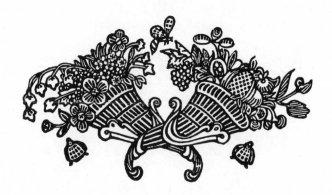

S tress and strain of daily life make us all vulnerable to headaches and nervous strain. After a hard day, it feels good to just relax with a warm cup of herbal tea and quiet our minds before tackling a busy evening.

Sometimes, nervous tension is one the causes of sleepless nights. There are times you may need help to get to sleep, but you should not rely on any drug or herb for long periods of time. They are to be used as a temporary help only. If the problem persists, you should see your physician for the cause of insomnia. If your health is good, it may be caused by an emotional problem.

Many times, we just do not need as many hours of sleep as we think we do. If everything is going pretty well in your life, but you just can't get to sleep, listen to your body. Maybe you need to stay up later then usual and attend to other things. Sometimes a sleepless night is a good time to get things done that you just don't have the time for during the day. There really is no need to worry if occasionally you are unable to get to sleep. There are studies that prove that staying up for 24 hours sometimes cures or helps depression. The time to worry is if you consistently cannot get to sleep and it interferes with your daily life. That is the time to contact your physician for help.

In addition to helping with headaches and sleeplessness, the recipes that follow are also good to use when you have a cold or the flu, as one of the symptoms is often a headache.

THIS ONE IS FOR HEADACHES, BUT ALSO IS AN ANTI-DEPRESSIVE: Pour 2 cups boiling water over 3 teaspoons dried primrose flowers and leaves. Let stand, covered, about 15 minutes. Strain and sweeten. Drink warm or hot. (Reheat as needed.) An older friend of mine has used this as an aid for over thirty years, so it must be very effective for her to have used it for so long.

ANOTHER ANTI-DEPRESSIVE: Put a handful of fresh chopped rosemary into a bottle of white wine. Let sit about 4 days. Strain and use by the tablespoon as needed. DELICIOUS! How could you stay depressed while taking so much pleasure in a taste sensation?

A FAVORITE FOR HEADACHES: Use 1 heaping teaspoon of dried chamomile flowers for each cup of boiling water. Steep 10 minutes. Strain and sweeten with honey. It's a good relaxer. *Caution:* Do not use if you suffer from ragweed allergies, as chamomile is in the same family. There are too many other herbs that you can substitute for you to take a chance of suffering from an allergic reaction. Great for those that can use it.

MAKE YOUR OWN PAIN KILLER: Soak 1/2 teaspoon of dried willow bark in 2 cups cold water overnight. Bring to a boil and simmer for 20 minutes. Strain, cool, and bottle. Dosage is 1/4 cup, to be sipped slowly as needed for pain.

This really does work. It can be added to juices or teas if you wish. Often, people are surprised that it works so fast. It's not so surprising when you remember that willow served as our first aspirin. Willow contains salicylates and was used as a pain killer until 1853. It was then taken from folk medicine and mass produced by a German chemist. In 1893, another German chemist, working for the Bayer Company, came up with the aspirin we now use. Aspirin's ingredients now come from coal-tar and petroleum products. We use about 100,000 tons of aspirin a year worldwide and it has become a favorite to treat many disorders or discomforts.

HEADACHE CAUSED BY MENTAL FATIGUE: Mix 1/2 teaspoon each of sage, peppermint, rosemary, and hops. Pour 2 cups boiling water over herb mixture and let steep 10 minutes. Add a pinch of ginger and sweeten. Drink warm before going to bed.

HEADACHES: Chop 1 cup fresh peppermint. Pour 2 cups boiling water over the herb and steep for 5 minutes. Strain and sweeten. Add lemon if desired. I use this one for the first twinge of a headache. Sometimes I can just think about getting a headache and that's enough of an excuse to sit and drink a cup. Very relaxing to me.

NERVOUS HEADACHES: Macerate 1 tablespoon of violet leaves and add to 1 cup of boiling water. Steep 10 minutes. Strain and sweeten with honey. This is said to quicken the intellect. I drink this a lot because of the vitamin A content. Knowing I am getting extra vitamins is enough of a kick for me, and I enjoy it that much more.

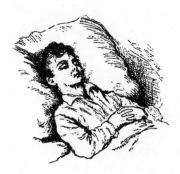

MIGRAINE HEADACHES: Many people suffer from migraines. From what I understand the pain can be terrific. Migraines can be precipitated by allergic hypersensitivity or emotional disturbances. Most people who suffer from the disorder come from a family background where over 50% of the family members suffer from the debilitating headaches. Rest in a darkened room is recommended. Try several of these remedies to find one that will work for you.

Put 10-15 elderberries in 1 cup of water. Mash berries and bring to a quick boil. Reduce heat and simmer for 10 minutes. Strain, sweeten and drink. This should be taken as soon as you feel a headache start on, as the analgesic effect is mild.

MIGRAINE HEADACHES: Mix equal parts of vinegar and water and bring to a boil. Inhale the fumes for several minutes. Repeat as needed.

MIGRAINE HEADACHES: This is a natural painkiller and is good for migraine headaches. Chop 1 tablespoon of Stinking Iris (*Iris foetidissima*) and add to 1 pint of water. Boil gently for 15 minutes. Strain and take up to 3 tablespoons per day. Has a slight laxative effect so you may want to weaken it further.

MIGRAINE HEADACHES: At the first sign of a headache, make a strong cup of coffee, adding 1 tablespoon of lemon juice. The caffeine in the coffee seems to help some migraine sufferers.

MIGRAINE HEADACHES: Put 2 tablespoons of dried nettle in 2 cups of milk. Simmer for 10 minutes. Strain and sweeten with honey. Drink while warm. Do not use if you show an allergic reaction to nettle. Substitute peppermint if need be. Test for allergic reaction by taking small sips the first time this recipe is tried. If no reaction or rash shows up, it would be safe to use.

MIGRAINE HEADACHES: Many people get relief from turning a hair dryer on medium setting at the first sign of a migraine headache and allowing the heat from the dryer to soothe their headache.

GOOD SEDATIVE: Mix together 1 tablespoon each of bee balm, hops, peppermint, chamomile, and crushed fennel seed. Add 1 tablespoon of the mixture to 1 cup boiling water. Steep 10 minutes and strain. Sweeten with honey. Drink 1/2 hour before bed.

NERVOUS TENSION: Vivid blue flowers are typical of many of the best nerve herbs and skullcap is one of them. Chop 1/2 cup of the leaves and flowers and add to 2 cups of boiling water. Steep 15 minutes and strain. Sweeten with honey and drink several cups a day. Can be used to treat epilepsy, convulsions, and any involuntary trembling of the limbs. Skullcap is also used during drug or alcohol withdrawal to lessen symptoms of withdrawal.

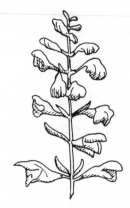

Skullcap (Scutellaria galericulata)

SKULLCAP BLEND: This is very good for nervous headaches. Mix 1 cup each of dried skullcap, sage and peppermint. To use, pour 1 cup boiling water over 1 teaspoon of herb mixture. Cover and let steep 10 minutes. Strain and sweeten. Drink warm as needed.

Skullcap is especially effective in dispelling headaches. It relaxes the whole system and is non-addictive.

CALM NERVES: Place 4-5 blossoms of cornflower in 1 cup of boiling water. Allow to steep 10 minutes. Strain and sweeten with honey. Used after strokes, cornflower tea is said to aid in returning the use of your limbs, if used regularly.

SEDATIVE: Cooked lettuce is a great relaxant. Lettuce tea is an even faster-acting sedative. Simply pour 1 cup boiling water over 1 cup shredded lettuce and steep 30 minutes. Strain and drink before bed. This really does work. It is one of the best relaxants that I know. Use to release tension or to help you if you suffer from insomnia. Great to use while a patient is recovering from any illness. It keeps them from getting restless and helps them get the rest they need in order for the body to finish the healing process.

HYSTERIA: To calm the patient, have them drink tea made from a bay leaf. Pour 1 cup boiling water over 2 bay leaves. Remove the leaves after steeping 10 minutes and sweeten with honey.

WOODRUFF OR SAGE TEA FOR HIGHLY AGITATED STATE:
Pour 1 cup boiling water over 1 teaspoon sweet woodruff or 1 teaspoon sage to bring immediate sense of calm. Let steep 15 minutes.
Strain and sweeten. I like the taste of the sweet woodruff tea better
than the sage. Both are effective and either can be used for the
same fast relief.

**NERVOUS ANXIETY THAT LEADS TO HEART PALPITA-
TIONS:** Pour 1 cup boiling water over 1 teaspoon of dried lemon
balm. Let steep 10 minutes. Strain and sweeten. This is a very
pleasant tasting tea. I like to add the lemon balm leaves to other
teas just for the taste alone. And the added benefits of being a great
relaxant are a plus in treating any illness.

SOOTHING BATH FOR TENSION HEADACHES: Put 1 ounce
each of mugwort, valerian, chamomile, and agrimony to 1 pint of
boiling water. Allow to simmer for 30 minutes. Strain and add to
bath water. Very good for aching muscles.

MILD SEDATIVE: Pour 1 pint boiling water over 1 teaspoon of
dried catnip. Cover and steep until cool. Flavor if desired. Strain
and sweeten. For children, give 1 tablespoon; adults get 2 tablespoons.

HOP SEDATIVE: Pour 1 quart boiling water over 1-1/2 teaspoons
dried hops flowers. Let steep, covered, 10 minutes. Strain and
sweeten. Add lemon juice if desired.

LAVENDER TEA: This is good for exhaustion and tension. Pour 1
cup boiling water over 1 teaspoon dried lavender flowers. Cover
and steep 15 minutes. Strain and sweeten. A good drink for after
work.
    This is a favorite of my daughter. She uses it quite frequently.

PEPPERMINT MIX: Mix 1 tablespoon each of dried peppermint
and bruised caraway seed. Pour 1 cup boiling water over 1 teaspoon of the mix and steep 15 minutes. Strain and sweeten with
honey.

This has the added benefits of soothing the stomach during upsets and relieving heartburn and indigestion. Also good to use during bouts of flu to settle the stomach.

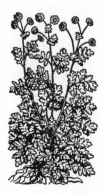

Feverfew (Chrysanthemum parthenium)

FOR TROUBLE GETTING TO SLEEP: Pour 1 pint of boiling water over 1 ounce of feverfew flowers. Cover and steep until cool. Strain and sweeten with honey. Drink cool.

TO INDUCE SLEEP: Mix 2 tablespoons dried peppermint with 1 tablespoon each of rosemary and sage. This really soothes the nerves and allows you to relax enough to go to sleep.

VALERIAN TEA: *Caution:* Take this only once a day (at bedtime, to induce sleep). Pour 1 pint boiling water over 1 teaspoon powdered valerian root. Cover and steep 10 minutes. Strain and sweeten. Add a pinch of mace as flavoring if desired. Drink warm.

Valerian is not a very pleasant smelling herb, but it is very effective. A friend of mine said she always makes sure that she is close to a bed when she makes this tea.

The valerian may be added to other, better tasting herbs and will be just as effective. Simply add the herb of your choice to the water along with the valerian.

BEE BALM SOOTHER: Pour 1 pint boiling water over 2 tablespoons of bee balm. Let steep for 15 minutes. Strain, sweeten and drink warm. Guaranteed to help put you to sleep.

SLEEP MIXTURE: Mix 1 tablespoon each of dried hop, chamomile, and lavender flowers, skullcap, and powdered valerian root. Put in size # 00 capsules. Take 2 capsules every couple of hours (not to exceed 6 capsules), shortly before you retire for the night. This should not be taken for longer then 2 days. If the problem persists after two days, please consult with your physician, to find out the reason for your inability to sleep. This is to be used only as a temporary measure.

ANISEED SLEEPER: Use 1 teaspoon of aniseed for each cup of water. Brew for about 20 minutes. Strain and sweeten. Induces sleep and aids in indigestion.

INSOMNIA: Eating an apple before bedtime seems to help put you to sleep.

INSOMNIA TREATMENT: Add 1 teaspoon pennyroyal herb to 1 cup boiling water. Let steep 15 minutes. Strain and sweeten. Drink warm before bed. *Caution:* Not to be used by pregnant women.

BUTTERMILK SLEEP AID: Drinking buttermilk before retiring aids in a good night's sleep. My mother and father both frequently had a glass of buttermilk before bed. I did not like the taste of buttermilk when I was younger, but I do now.

SLEEP AID: Heat 1 cup of milk and add 2 tablespoons of honey and 2 teaspoons of lemon juice. Drink 1/2 hour before retiring.

OATMEAL SLEEP AID: Make oatmeal as you normally would, but add milk enough to make a thin gruel. Drink this before bed as a help in getting to sleep. This is a very relaxing way to get children to sleep. It seems to soothe them and make their tummies feel warm and full. It is also good to use during bouts of illness, as it does soothe the stomach and settle upsets, while being nutritious. Make it very special by adding sugar and a pinch of ground cinnamon. Children really do love this. It helps restless children get a good night's sleep.

RESTLESSNESS AT BEDTIME: Put several passion flower blooms into 1 cup of boiling water. Steep 10 minutes. Add honey and drink before retiring.

YAWN YOURSELF TO SLEEP: If you suffer from insomnia, simply practice yawning and before you know it you will be asleep. My husband didn't believe this until he tried it.

INSOMNIA IN OLDER PERSONS: Put 1/2 cup of violet flowers in 1 cup of boiling water. Cover and let stand at least 24 hours. Add 1-1/2 cups of sugar and simmer 15 minutes. Strain and drink before bed. This can be taken nightly, if desired. It helps you to relax as well as giving you extra vitamins. Children also enjoy this tea. It helps them to get a good night's sleep and supplies the extra vitamins that all children need for good eye sight.

TO INDUCE SLEEP: Mix together 2 tablespoons chamomile, 2 tablespoons skullcap, 1 teaspoon goldenseal, 2 teaspoons elder flower, 1/2 teaspoon peppermint powder and 1 tablespoon pennyroyal. Add mixture to 2 cups of water. Bring to a boil and then reduce to a simmer. Simmer until liquid is reduced by half. Bottle and label. Dosage is 1-2 tablespoons to one cup of hot water. Sweeten to taste. Take at bedtime to induce sleep.

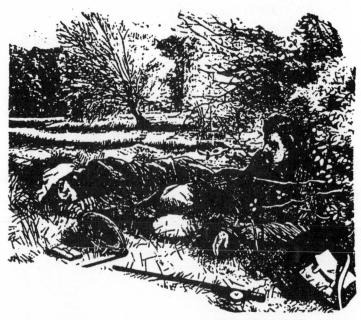

·9·

Diuretics and Bowel Complaints

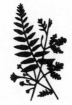

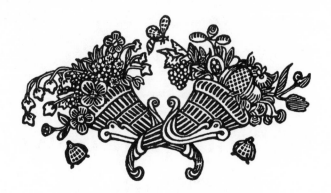

I f you keep to a healthy diet you should not have too much trouble with your bowels. A diet with a good balance of fruits and vegetables helps to regulate the bowels. Some people think that having a lot of bran in their diet works well. That's true, but, eating a lot of bran will not help you if you do not take in plenty of water to help it work.

A good exercise program also helps. Keeping the back and stomach muscles strong goes a long way to helping you feel good and keeping you and your bowels healthy. Walking is still the best way to get exercise. The whole family can get into the habit of walking and everybody benefits.

Some of my kids' best childhood memories are of the walks we took. We always headed out to the woods, with a stop in the garden to pick our lunch. We even had a dog that would go to the garden and eat peas right off the vine. The kids got in the habit of eating raw vegetables in this way and enjoyed the walks so much that they continue the practice.

Kids love to walk, even in the rain. Remember how much fun you had as a child when you were caught out in the rain? I loved to play in the rain when I was younger. I taught my kids a game that I played when I was young. We called the game "running in the wind." We would play it right before a big storm. Even today I run for the front porch so I can watch a storm coming on. I guess my love of nature came about because I was able to participate in the changes of the seasons.

Learn to enjoy all the seasons by taking walks all year round. Your health really does benefit and it's a good way to learn to identify the wild herbs. Take a good herbal reference book with you when you go and you will find all kinds of treasures.

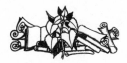

Some people, for one reason or another, seem to be prone to kidney or bladder infections. It does help to use diuretics to flush the kidneys every once in a while, even if you are not troubled in this way. Diuretics increase the flow of urine. The body rids itself of poisons through the urinary system. You should drink plenty of water to help it do this. To help you, there are many herbs that are good diuretics. You will want to try several until you find the one that suits you. Also, it doesn't hurt to fast while you are treating either the urinary tract or the bowels.

As you look over these recipes, remember that herbs are not intended to take the place of your family physician, nor are they an overnight cure for ills. It takes much more time to heal then the duration of an illness.

BURDOCK SEED DIURETIC: Add 1 teaspoon crushed burdock seeds to 1 pint of boiling water. Steep covered for 30 minutes. Strain, and drink in order to flush kidneys and bladder. Good to use when troubled by kidney stones.

THYME TREATMENT: Thyme is a good astringent so it will work to clean the kidneys and bladder. Pour 1 cup boiling water over 1 teaspoon of thyme. Let sit for 15 minutes. Strain and sweeten with honey. Drink 1 cup a day for 1 week.

TO TONE UP THE KIDNEYS: Chop several leaves of aloe vera and put into a pint of water. Place in the refrigerator and drink a little every day to tone up the kidneys. This can also be used for headaches. Many people swear by this remedy and drink the juice of aloe vera on a daily basis, as it keeps the whole body toned up.

DIURETIC: To make a good diuretic, pour 1 pint of boiling water over a handful of borage leaves. Let sit for 15 minutes. Strain and sweeten if desired. Drink several cups daily for 2 days.

USE OFTEN TO FLUSH THE KIDNEYS: Firmly pack fresh parsley (stems and all) into a one-cup measuring cup. Pour 1 quart of boiling water over the parsley. Let steep until cool. Strain and refrigerate. Sweeten as desired. Reheat as needed. Drink several cups for 2 days. I do this several times during the summer when the parsley is new in the garden. I use a lot of parsley when I cook and I dry at least 3 quarts yearly.

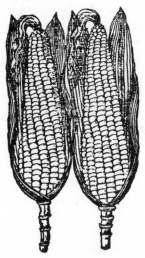

Corn (Zea mays)

CORN SILK DIURETIC: This works to clear the kidneys rapidly. Pour 2 cups boiling water over 1 tablespoon corn silk. Let simmer 5 minutes. Strain, sweeten and drink as much as you like for 2 days. I give this to my husband, as I consider it good for the prostate too. I dry plenty of corn silk when I can corn, so it it is on hand when I need it later on in the winter. This is one of the easier herbs to get and dry. You can simply save the corn silk from the times you husked corn for corn-on-the-cob.

FENNEL FLUSH: Pour 1/2 pint boiling water over 1 teaspoon ✓ bruised fennel seed. Let steep until cool. Sweeten to taste. Drink 3 cups a day for 2 days.

DIURETIC: Pour 2 cups boiling water over 2 teaspoons dried meadowsweet flowers and leaves. Let steep, covered, 15 minutes. Strain and sweeten. Drink 1 cup after meals for 1 week.

GOOD DIURETIC: Pour 2 pints boiling water over 1 ounce of bruised mustard seed and 2 ounces freshly chopped horseradish root. Cover and steep 4-5 hours. Strain and bottle. Dosage is 3 tablespoons 3 times daily for 2 days.

DIURETIC: Do not use this one for over 2 days as it is very strong (and effective). Chop 2 pounds of parsley and add to 1 quart of milk. Place in an oven at low heat (about 150-175 degrees). Take out when liquid is reduced to about half. Cool thoroughly and strain. Take 1 tablespoon every 2 hours for 1 day. Skip 1 day and repeat the next. Use this if you suffer from repeated kidney or bladder infections. Clears up the problem fast.

CORN SILK DIURETIC: Add 1 ounce of corn silk to 1 pint of boiling water. Allow to steep 15 minutes. Drink throughout the day for sudden cystitis. Works pretty fast. Use for 1 day.

CYSTITIS: Put 1 teaspoon fresh parsley in 1 cup of boiling water ✓ and steep 15 minutes. Strain and sweeten. Drink several cups a day for 2 days.

AIDS URINATION: Pour 1 cup boiling water over 1 teaspoon tarragon and steep 15 minutes. Strain and sweeten. Drink several cups daily for 2 days.

TREATMENT FOR KIDNEY AILMENTS: Core and peel a pear, then puree it in the blender. Place the pear mixture in a pan and add 1 pint of boiled water. Stir in 1/4 cup of honey. Drink often during the day for 2 days.

KIDNEY STONES: To help pass kidney stones, make a tea using 1/4 teaspoon of dried parsley, 1 cup boiled water, 1 tablespoon lemon juice and 1 tablespoon olive oil. Drink every day for at least a week.

TREATMENT FOR URINARY TRACT PROBLEMS: Put 2 teaspoons of sweet basil in 1 cup of boiling water. Steep 10 minutes. Drink this 2 times daily for 2 days.

URINARY TRACT TREATMENT: Put 1 tablespoon each of heartsease (pansy) and young blackberry leaves in 2 cups of boiling water and steep for 15 minutes. Strain and sweeten. Drink several cups daily for 2 days.

BLADDER HELP: Pour 1 cup of water over 3 teaspoons crushed rose hips. Bring to a boil and boil gently for 3 minutes. Strain and drink 4 times a day for 2 days.

ONE OF THE BEST WAYS TO CLEAR UP KIDNEY OR BLADDER INFECTIONS: Do not drink any other liquids except water during this treatment.

Get or make plenty of cranberry juice. Drink it the first thing in the morning and the last thing at night. Drink it as often as possible during the day, along with plenty of water in between the cranberry juice. If the infection is not too bad, it should be cleared by next morning. In more severe cases, it may take several days.

If you are prone to infections of the kidney or bladder, it would do you good to make a habit of drinking cranberry juice at least once a day. This really is one of the best habits to have. Cranberries are a good remedy to use for many different illnesses. They do contain a substance that dilates the bronchial tubes and are used by asthmatics. They are good for removing toxins from the blood and are very effective in treating liver problems. They also contain diuretic properties and are an excellent way to treat most kidney problems.

CUCUMBER HELP FOR KIDNEY PROBLEMS: Cucumbers are among the best of treatments for kidney or bladder problems. Drinking cucumber juice alone or added to other vegetable juices is an excellent way to treat and correct kidney problems. Adding cucumber juice to carrot juice is a great remedy to prepare when there is an excess retention of uric acid in the system. Cucumbers are also used to correct high or low blood pressure because of their high potassium content.

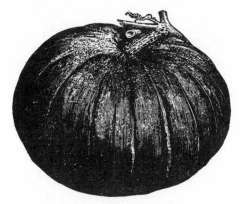

Pumpkin (Cucurbita pepo)

PROSTATE GLAND HELPER: Pumpkin seeds are known for their use in restoring the healthy functioning of the prostate gland. They should be eaten daily by men who suffer from problems in that area.

A tea may be made for those suffering from inflammation of the bladder and the prostate. Add 4 ounces of whole pumpkin seed to 1 quart of water and simmer 30 minutes. Do not strain, but allow to cool before drinking. Drink several glasses a day, as needed, for treatment and for the pain. This is a really a good way to treat any problems dealing with the prostate. I know many men who use this tea at least once a week.

FASTING: To keep the body flushed of toxins, fast one day a month, drinking fruit juices only.

FLUSH OUT FAT: Mix together 2 large carrots, 1 cup fresh parsley, 1-1/2 cups chopped spinach, 1 cup freshly chopped comfrey leaves, a couple of stalks of celery, 1 cup green beans and 2-1/2 cups of water in a large blender. Add ginger to taste, refrigerate.

Drink as often as desired. Really flushes out the fat if used on a regular basis. Very high energy food.

BEDWETTING REMEDY: Allow the child to drink 4 ounces of cranberry juice before going to bed. Adults should drink 8 ounces. This helps a lot of people.

BEDWETTING REMEDY: Put 1/2 teaspoon of Epsom salts in any liquid and drink after your supper. This really does help.

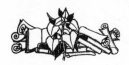

During some illnesses we have to contend with diarrhea. Here are some recipes to help with that problem.

DIARRHEA CONTROL: When blackberries are in season, pick plenty so you can put up plenty of good juice. When you can the berries, cold pack them so the juice is extracted. Then you have the use of the berries after draining off the juice.

Blackberry juice is very good for treating diarrhea in children. Give a glassful every couple of hours as needed. You will probably want to sweeten the juice a little. My kids always loved this and we would drink it just for the heck of it, even when not needed.

I really miss having the kids pick berries with me, because this was one of our best times together. We always had a lot of fun. Some of the kids come over to go picking now—and I really enjoy that—but it seems that small children can make any situation more fun. Even bugs can create a fascinating conversation. Kids come up with the funniest notions about life. You learn a lot just by listening to them.

TREATING DIARRHEA IN CHILDREN: Children dehydrate very quickly by losing fluid and salts in the body due to diarrhea, fever, and vomiting. It is important to replace the fluids through any liquid the child will drink, and to continue to feed them the liquid.

Prepare the following rehydration drink and give at the onset of diarrhea. Mix together 1 teaspoon of table salt, 8 teaspoons sugar, and add to 5 cups of water. (If you have time, sterilize the water by boiling it, but be sure to cool it before giving it to the child.) Give 1 cup each time the child has a bowel movement, half of that for a smaller child. Spoon-feed the babies. Let the child drink as much as they want. You can stop giving it as soon as the child stops having loose bowel movements or loses desire for the rehydration drink.

Seek help if the child displays symptoms of dehydration, if there is severe vomiting, or if they will not drink. For babies, you should seek help immediately. The rehydration solution is for emergency use only; it is just to tide you over until you can seek medical help. Deaths from dehydration are common, so do not hesitate to contact your physician.

PLANTAIN INFUSION: Plantain is easy to find, so dry plenty of it. It has many uses. The ribbed plantain is the best for medicinal use, so try to collect only that kind.

This recipe is good for treating diarrhea. Pour 1 cup boiling water over 2 ounces dried plantain leaves. Cover and steep 20 minutes. Strain and sweeten. Drink in 1/2 cup doses every 2 hours until relief is obtained.

COMFREY CONTROL FOR DIARRHEA: Heat 1 quart of milk until hot. Add 1/2 ounce of comfrey root. Steep 15 minutes. Strain. Drink a glass every hour until relief is obtained.

DIARRHEA CONTROL: Heat 1 cup of milk. Add 1 teaspoon of nutmeg. Stir well and drink warm. Do this every hour until relief is obtained. Honey may be added if desired.

DIARRHEA CONTROL: Mix 1 cup blackberry juice and 1 tablespoon wild geranium, 1 tablespoon shepherd's purse, 1 tablespoon sweet fern, and 1 teaspoon of ginger. Boil for 10 minutes. Cool and strain. Drink 1/2 cup every hour, or after every bowel movement. Do not eat solids until diarrhea is cleared up. Then start to eat on a light diet.

DIARRHEA: Put a pinch of allspice in 1 cup of warm water. Add honey and drink after every bowel movement.

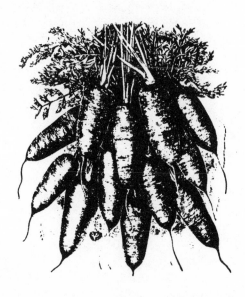

Carrots (Daucus carota)

CARROTS FOR DIARRHEA: Cook 1 pound of carrots in as little water as possible. Cook until soft. When done, puree in the blender. Keep refrigerated and take 1/4 cup every 30 minutes until relief is obtained.

DIARRHEA CONTROL: Boil 2/3 cup of white or brown rice in 1 quart of water for 15 minutes. Strain and sip the resulting liquid. Should get relief in a couple of hours.

DIARRHEA: Peel, core and puree an apple in the blender. Grate if you do not have a blender. Give 1 apple every 2 hours, while withholding all other food during treatment.

APPLE DRINK FOR DIARRHEA: Simmer 1 pared apple in 1 cup of milk until very soft. Put apple/milk mixture in the blender and blend until smooth. Drink 1/2 cup after every bowel movement until relief is obtained.

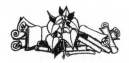

Sometimes the problem is just the opposite: constipation can be very uncomfortable. Treat it as soon as possible. However, do not use a laxative on a very weak person or on one who is recovering from a debilitating illness. Children also should not receive a laxative. It would be better to use a suppository on small children and a mild enema on older children. I used to cut a small sliver of hand soap and use it as a suppository for my children when they were babies. It worked well.

CASTOR OIL TREATMENT: This works quickly, but again, do not use on someone who is in a weakened condition. It's guaranteed to work. Soak a flannel cloth in warm castor oil. I put mine in a cake pan and pour the oil over the cloth, then place it in the oven until warmed through. Place on the small of the back and cover to keep warm. Keep on at least 15 minutes. Do once a day until bowels have moved satisfactorily.

ALOE VERA LAXATIVE: To sterilize the water, boil it and then cool it. Peel the aloe vera. Put the green peelings and the water in a closed jar. (The juice is not the part used for a laxative, it's the sap between the skin and the pulp.) Place in the refrigerator and drink 1 cup twice a week to regulate bowels. The strength is determined by the amount of aloe vera placed in the water. Start with several leaves, and add until desired strength is reached.

LAXATIVE: Take 2 tablespoons of black strap molasses before retiring to bed. This does work. Add to a glass of milk or juice if desired to improve the flavor.

CLOVE LAXATIVE: Pour 1 cup boiling water over 1 teaspoon of whole cloves. Cover and steep overnight. Strain the next morning and drink while cool.

APPLE JUICE LAXATIVE: Mix together 1/2 cup of apple juice and 1/2 cup of olive oil. Drink before going to bed.

PRUNE LAXATIVE: Pour boiling water over several prunes and allow to soak overnight. Add honey if you desire sweetening. Eat the prunes and drink the liquid.

REGULATE BOWELS TO PREVENT CONSTIPATION: Put 2 teaspoons corn meal in 1 cup of cold water every morning and drink daily. Helps to regulate bowels.

REGULATE BOWELS: Mix 1 teaspoon each of lemon juice and olive oil. Take on a daily basis.

HEMORRHOID TREATMENT: Mix 8 tablespoons willow bark, 3 tablespoons of horse weed, 6 tablespoons red oak bark, 4 tablespoons pilewort, and 4 tablespoons sage. Add 1/2 teaspoon of this herb mixture to 1 pint boiling water. Let stand, covered, until cool. Strain and use as a rectal enema before going to bed.

TREATING COLITIS: Colitis can become a serious disorder. It is an inflammation of the colon. Symptoms include watery stools with mucus and pus in the stool. There is abdominal tenderness and pain along with swelling. Dip a flannel cloth in apple cider vinegar and place on the abdomen. Cover with plastic and allow to stay in place for at least 4 hours. This should provide relief.

TREATING COLITIS: Mix 2 cups of Epsom salts in 1 pint of water. Saturate a flannel cloth in the salt solution and place over the abdomen. Keep warm with a heating pad or water bottle for 3-4 hours.

·10·

Blood Disorders, Wounds and Arthritis

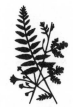

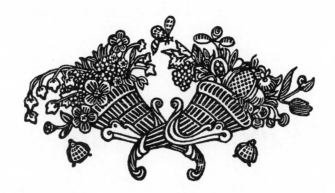

What do blood disorders, wounds, and arthritis all have in common? They are all linked to the health of the blood and the circulatory system. And they are all conditions that have a history of good herbal remedies behind them.

All the body's cells must be supplied with nutrients and oxygen constantly. The blood carries oxygen through the circulatory system. A good diet is important to keep the blood built up and to ensure that there is no deficiency of necessary minerals and vitamins.

These vitamins and minerals help keep the blood healthy, so it can do its job. One of its jobs is to clot when there's a wound. Wounds depend on the clotting ability of the blood to stop bleeding.

Good circulation is important when you have arthritis. Exercise can help. It is important to exercise on a daily basis. If you are afraid exercising will be painful, try taking a warm bath before attempting to do any exercises. Check with your doctor if you are concerned about exercising.

There are many different types of arthritis and none are easy to live with. There is a type of arthritis that is associated with psoriasis. Bursitis is also a form of arthritis.

The studies done on rheumatoid arthritis have caused many to believe that the pathological changes to the joints are caused by an antigen-antibody reaction that is still not understood. If the condition is severe, bed rest is important for a short time. When the period of inflammation is gone, it is important that you get up and resume as normal a lifestyle as possible. Exercise is important because you must maintain muscle strength and keep the range of motion of the affected joints.

High blood pressure is a common disorder and a silent killer. It should be taken seriously. While trying the herbs as a remedy, it is important that you continue any medication that your physician has prescribed for you. I do want to caution you to continue with any treatment that your physician is using in treating your high blood pressure. Perhaps you could work with him or her to supplement your treatment with some of the more natural treatments.

Physicians, too, can learn a lot from you about respecting nature and using it to their advantage. The more discerning physicians are becoming more aware every day of natural methods and are relating this to their treatment of patients. Many doctors are finding that there are alternatives to prescribing drugs. By studying the natural methods, they have realized there are many different ways to deal with human illness.

You could check with your doctor to see if he or she approves of some of these ways to help with high blood pressure: Watch your diet, exercise regularly, cut down on salt intake, and keep your stress level low. It doesn't hurt to stop and smell the roses and it wouldn't hurt to start a meditation program to help you cope with stress.

I am a firm believer that stress is our number one killer. I also believe that learning to cooperate with nature and learning to love the quiet times can be a lifesaver. If we but study some of the laws of nature, we could learn to use those laws in our own lives. The trees bend with the wind in order not to break. We can use this advice in our own life. If we learn to bend when times are rough, we can ride out the hard times, too.

The changes of the seasons teach us that we, too, have changes in our life. Learn to appreciate them. Learn that out of destruction can come great blessings and new beginnings. Everything has a season and time for being—it's a natural law.

We can learn patience by living with this law. We learn that the less we fight against something and the more we cooperate, the easier life gets. I relate this to gardening. We all fight the weeds so hard that we lose the pleasure of the garden, and nature becomes an enemy. Learn about some of the weeds and you find that they, too, have a lot to offer us.

We can learn more about some natural methods to take care of our gardens. We can become protective of the food chain and fight to stop some of the more harmful methods now in use to control nature. Even the insects have a place in the food chain. We can learn to respect insects, animals and people—along with Mother Nature. We can learn that to give thanks is helpful—even to plants. Life just seems to get much easier when we stop fighting and start living.

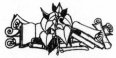

BLOOD PRESSURE TREATMENT: Cayenne pepper is very good for lowering blood pressure. You will see results when next you have your pressure read. It is good for the whole system and is a great stimulant.

Add 1 teaspoon cayenne pepper to 1 cup of hot water. Drink once daily. Another way to take it is to fill #00 capsules with cayenne pepper and take 2 capsules twice daily.

HIGH BLOOD PRESSURE TREATMENT: Take 1000 mg of calcium daily for 8 weeks. This should reduce high blood pressure substantially.

HIGH BLOOD PRESSURE: Mix equal parts of chamomile, mint, and tag alder. Make as follows: Simmer 1 ounce of the herb mixture in 1 pint of water for 20 minutes. Strain and drink tepid. Drink 1/2 cup 3 times daily.

HIGH BLOOD PRESSURE: Remove the seeds from 1 pound of hawthorn berries and soak overnight in about 80 ounces of water. Bring to a boil the next day and boil for 10 minutes. Cool, strain and drink 2-3 cups per day. Said to lower blood pressure.

BLOOD PRESSURE CAPSULES: I have made these for my son-in-law. He took them with his prescription and his blood pressure did decrease for the first time in several months.

For this recipe, use powdered herbs if possible, as it will save you time. Mix together 1 tablespoon each of nettle, mint, elder, and chamomile. Then add 1 teaspoon each of lobelia and valerian root. Place in #00 capsules and take 1 daily. Makes about 71 capsules.

HIGH BLOOD PRESSURE TEA: Mix 1 tablespoon each of tag alder, chamomile, and peppermint. Pour 1 cup boiling water over 1 teaspoon of the herb mixture. Steep 15 minutes. Strain and sweeten with honey before drinking.

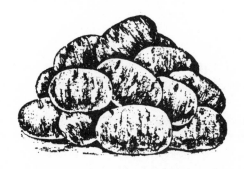

Potatoes (Solanum tuberosum)

BLOOD PRESSURE TREATMENT: Wash 5-6 potatoes and peel. Place the peelings in 2 cups of water and boil for 15 minutes, covered. Steep until cool and strain. Drink 2 cups of this liquid every day. Said to bring high blood pressure down to normal.

The Irish sure got their money's worth with the potatoes. It is used to cure many different illnesses as well as serving as a staple in our diet. I think that it is amazing that so many different cultures found so many uses for the common everyday plants that are all around us.

HIGH BLOOD PRESSURE TREATMENT: Put the juice from a lemon in a glass of warm water and add 1 tablespoon of honey. Mix well and drink daily.

HIGH BLOOD PRESSURE TREATMENT: Grind up 1/4 cup of watermelon seeds and add to 1 pint of water. Boil gently for 15 minutes. Strain and add honey to sweeten. Watermelon has long been used as treatment for high blood pressure.

HIGH BLOOD TREATMENT: Meadowsweet is very high in magnesium and iron. It can be used for all blood disorders. Put 1 ounce of meadowsweet in 3/4 pint of boiling water. Allow to steep 10 minutes. Strain and drink several times a day.

REGULATE BLOOD PRESSURE: Prepare a tea from leaves and stems of hyssop to help regulate high or low blood pressure. Place a handful of chopped leaves and stems of hyssop in 1 pint of boiling water. Steep 10 minutes. Strain and sweeten with honey. Drink twice daily.

HIGH BLOOD PRESSURE TREATMENT: Combine a small handful of chopped primrose leaves and flowers to a salad daily. Can also use to make tea. Add about 1/4 cup primrose leaves and flowers to 1 cup boiling water. Steep 10 minutes. Strain and sweeten. Drink with meals.

Caution: **Diabetics and hypoglycemics should not take calendula in any form internally. It drops the blood sugar level drastically and is potentially very dangerous.**

TREATMENT FOR HIGH BLOOD SUGAR: Put 1 teaspoon of dried and crushed blueberry leaves *(vaccinium spp.)* in 1 cup of boiling water. Steep 15 minutes. Strain and drink every 6 hours.

DIABETES: Diabetics will benefit from drinking strawberry tea. Place 4-5 fresh leaves in 1 cup of boiling water. Steep 15 minutes. Strain and drink.

DIABETES: Diabetics are said to benefit from drinking tea made from wild carrots (Queen Anne's Lace). Place several blossoms in 1 cup of boiling water and steep 10 minutes. Strain and drink several cups a day.

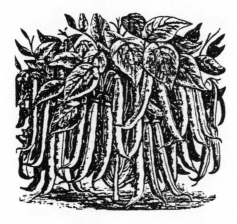

Green Beans (Phaseolus spp.)

DIABETES: A friend of mine (who was diabetic) gave me this information about 10 years ago. Her physician had given her this recipe to use. She lived to be in her eighties, so I guess it worked.

The skins of the green bean pods are said to contain substances that are related to insulin. She placed about 1 quart of green bean pods in about 4 quarts of water and cooked them until soft. She strained the pods from the liquid and drank 3 cups a day with her meals. One cup was said to equal 1 unit of insulin.

BEE POLLEN TREATMENT FOR ANEMIA: Bee pollen is a biological stimulant that increases the red blood cells in bone marrow. You should take 1 teaspoon of bee pollen daily to treat anemia.

TREATMENT FOR ANEMIA: You should eat plenty of liver, but if you do not like it, you should take desiccated liver tablets daily. Eating plenty of green vegetables is also of great help.

Believe it or not, red wine can build the blood as well as anything can. My physician put me on a daily glass of red wine years ago after I had contracted a severe staph infection while in the hospital. My blood count had dropped so drastically that I almost didn't make it. My weight had gone down from 98 pounds to 78 pounds. I am only 5 feet tall so at that time in my life 98 pounds was normal for me. The 78 pounds was horrible. I looked like a walking skeleton. After my three weeks in the hospital, I started on the wine therapy and it did pick up my appetite as well as build up my blood count. And I enjoyed my afternoon pick-me-up.

BLACK STRAP MOLASSES ANEMIA TREATMENT: Black-strap molasses has more iron then liver. Try to have 1/3 cup daily. Mix with milk or use for sweetener if possible.

ANEMIA TREATMENT: Mix 2 teaspoons each of apple cider vinegar and blackstrap molasses with water or tea to strengthen the blood.

BLOOD BUILDER: Put 1 teaspoon each of dried comfrey, fenugreek seed, and dandelion in 2 cups of boiling water. Steep 10 minutes. Strain and add honey as sweetener. Drink after meals.

BLOOD BUILDER: Add 1 ounce of ground orange peel, 1/2 teaspoon of ground ginger and 1 ounce of chamomile to 2 cups of boiling water. Steep until cool. Strain, and add to 1 cup of brandy. Dosage is 1/2 cup in the morning and again in the evening.

PAINFUL MENSTRUATION: During your menstrual cycle, drink several glasses of red raspberry juice daily to prevent cramps and pain. I plan on planting several dozen of the red raspberry vines in the back of one of my herb beds. I plan on having plenty of raspberries on hand to give away, because I know many young women who could benefit from them. Besides, I love eating the berries.

MENSTRUAL CRAMPS: Mix 1 ounce each of cramp bark, skullcap, and blue cohosh. Add 1 teaspoon of cinnamon. Place in a quart of warm wine. Steep for several days. Strain and take 1 tablespoon doses several times a day for cramps.

CRAMPING DURING MENSTRUATION: Pour 1 cup of boiling water over 1 tablespoon of dried raspberry leaves. Cover and allow to steep 15 minutes. Strain and sweeten. Drink warm several times during the day.

OVERLY HEAVY MENSTRUATION: Put 1 tablespoon of chopped shepherd's purse in 1 pint of boiling water and allow to steep 30 minutes. Strain and put 1 tablespoon of the liquid in 1/3 cup of water and drink several times a day. This relieves cramps and helps to regulate the flow.

FOR HEAVY MENSTRUATION: Strawberry leaves were traditionally used to prevent miscarriages and hemorrhages. Place a small handful of fresh strawberry leaves in 1 pint of boiling water and steep 15 minutes. Strain and sweeten. Drink several times daily if your period is heavy. Supplies the body with needed iron and is good to treat anemia.

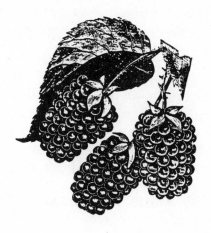

Raspberries (Rubas strigosus)

HELP THROUGH MENOPAUSE: Raspberry leaf tea is an excellent way to get more minerals in your system and is helpful to most female problems. Aids in menstrual discomfort as well as easing the symptoms of menopause. Put 10 fresh raspberry leaves in 1 cup of boiling water and allow to simmer 10 minutes. Strain and sweeten. You should drink several cups at this strength every day. Also calms the nerves when jittery.

GINGER HELP: Fresh ground ginger stops the formation of blood clots. Grind 1/2 teaspoon of fresh ginger and add to 1 cup of boiling water. Sweeten with honey and drink hot.

TO INCREASE THE BODY'S ABILITY TO DISSOLVE BLOOD CLOTS: English scientists are advocating the eating of fried onions to help the body dissolve and prevent blood clots.

AN OLD REMEDY TO STOP THE FLOW OF BLOOD FROM WOUNDS: Gather up cobwebs and roll in a ball. Save these to apply to wounds that are bleeding, as it stops the blood quickly. It would take a diligent person to gather up cobwebs, but the knowledge might come in handy some day.

TO STAUNCH THE FLOW OF BLOOD: Bruise a handful of lemon balm leaves and stems. Apply to the injury. Bind up with a clean bandage and leave on until the blood flow stops.

TO STOP BLEEDING: Apply witch hazel directly to cuts and scrapes. It is important that you care for cuts, scrapes or sores immediately, to prevent infection and to begin rapid healing.

TO STOP BLEEDING IMMEDIATELY: Dry the inner spores of the puff-ball mushroom. Apply directly to the wound. This will cause the blood to clot quickly.

Caution: Use care in storing this, as the powder was used in early photography as flash powder and is highly explosive. This is one of the best methods I know to stem the flow of blood. I plan on renewing my supply this year. It keeps forever and you need only gather it as needed (every couple of years or so).

ST. JOHN'S WORT REMEDY: St. John's wort was often given to patients recovering from surgery because it has painkilling properties and it helped to prevent hemorrhages. Scientists are now testing it for use in the fight against AIDS. It strengthens the immune system and is also used in cancer treatment.

Chop 1/2 cup of the leaves and stems and add to 1 pint of boiling water. Allow to steep for 15 minutes. Strain and drink several cups a day. *Caution:* This should not be taken for longer than one week.

POULTICE HELP: When applying a liquid poultice to injuries, it is helpful to soak a piece of bread in the liquid and place the bread on the area needed. The bread molds itself to the injured site and keeps the herbal liquid in constant contact with the injury.

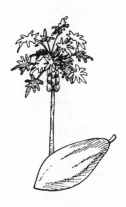

Papaya (Carica papaya)

CLEANING INFECTED WOUNDS: Apply papaya juice to the wound that has become infected. First wash the wound with the juice, then allow it to dry on the wound naturally.

TREATING INFLAMED WOUNDS: Put a handful of mallow root and leaves in a quart of water. Strain and use as wash for wounds that are inflamed. Wash the wound at least twice daily, putting on a fresh bandage each time.

TREATING INFECTED WOUNDS: Place several comfrey leaves (also called blackwort) and several cloves of garlic in the blender. Add a little honey and blend well. Spread the mixture on a slice of bread and place on the infected wound. Bandage and repeat several times a day, cleaning the wound each time before applying a fresh poultice.

POULTICE FOR WOUNDS: Bruise a handful of fresh oak leaves and apply directly to the wound. Cover with a warm cloth.

POULTICE: Put a handful of honeysuckle leaves in a pint of water and bring to a boil. Lower heat and simmer for 15 minutes. Use to wash the wound and use the liquid as a poultice.

COMBAT INFLAMMATION OF WOUNDS: Bruise plantain leaves and bind to wound after cleansing.

POULTICE FOR SWOLLEN GLANDS AND BOILS: Macerate a small handful of violet leaves and apply to the area. Keep warm by covering with flannel cloth. People often ask what macerate means. I tell them it means to mush up the plant. The dictionary says it means to soften and I don't know how else to describe it rather than to tell you to mush up the leaves.

POULTICE FOR WOUNDS: Apply fresh cut papaya slices to the wound and bandage overnight. Will clear up the infection and speed healing.

POULTICE FOR WOUNDS: Pound the roots and leaves of honeysuckle and apply them to a clean cloth. Apply to the wound and bind it up.

SORES OR WOUNDS: Use aloe vera for sores to prevent infection. Place a split aloe vera leaf over the area and cover with a clean bandage. Leave on overnight. This is good for any skin injury.

PUNCTURE WOUNDS: Put 2 tablespoons of St. John's wort in 1 cup of boiling water. Allow to steep until cool. Use this to clean the wound and allow the liquid to dry naturally on the wound. Apply a bandage that has been saturated with the herbal liquid to the wound. Keep the area clean and soak area in the liquid if possible. Will provide pain relief and promote healing.

TREATMENT OF INFECTED PUNCTURE WOUNDS: Place a piece of moldy bacon fat on the wound and bandage overnight. It will draw the infection from the wound.

STOP PAIN OF PUNCTURE WOUNDS: Pour kerosene on the wound immediately after the injury. It will take the soreness and pain from the wound.

I use this method often. I go barefoot most of the time and with all of the construction that is goes on around here, I have had quite a few injuries. When we were first clearing the land to build our house, I was up here alone clearing some bushes. I had a rake with me that I was using. Because I was not being careful and was not watching what I was doing, I stepped backwards onto the rake. It went clear through the foot and I had an awful time pulling the rake back through the foot and shoe. If I had not had the kerosene to pour on the foot I would have had to stay off my feet for weeks. As it was, I never had to stop using the foot; I only had to hobble around for several days. Kerosene does help take most of the soreness out.

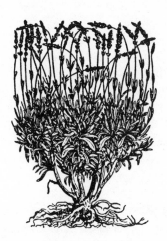

Lavender (Lavendula officinale)

SORES OR ULCERS: Use an antiseptic or astringent to wash sores and ulcers. Grind 2 tablespoons each of lavender flowers and cinnamon. Add this to a pint of ethyl alcohol. Close tightly and allow to steep for 2 weeks. Strain, bottle and label. Always keep this on hand. Great for when kids get scrapes, cuts and scratches.

SKIN ULCERS AND VARICOSE VEINS: The major use of calendula was to treat varicose veins, although it is very useful to treat skin ulcers that are associated with varicose veins. Place 1 cup of calendula leaves, fresh or dried, into an earthenware bowl. Pour 2 cups of boiling water over the leaves. Steep for 30 minutes. Strain and use directly on the ulcer as a wash.

VARICOSE VEINS: Aloe vera juice can also be used to treat varicose veins. Apply the juice directly to the area. Said to be very soothing.

VARICOSE TREATMENT: Crush 1 handful of violet leaves and flowers and pour 1 cup boiling water over the violets. Steep until cool. Use as a poultice to relieve pain. This is also a good wash for any open ulcers. Soak a bandage in the liquid and leave on overnight. Replace in the morning. Continue the treatment until improvement is noticed.

VARICOSE TREATMENT: Tansy is good to use to treat varicose veins. Make a tea using 1 teaspoon of tansy to each cup of boiling water. Steep 10 minutes and strain. Apply the tea externally to varicose veins and bruises.

CIRCULATORY PROBLEMS: Add 1 teaspoon cayenne pepper to 1 cup hot water. Drink daily. Apply cayenne pepper liberally to your food.

LEG ULCERS: Put 4 leaves of comfrey in the blender and add 1/4 cup of water. Blend well and use as a poultice daily. After you have removed the poultice, wash the area gently and apply the oil from 3 broken capsules of goldenseal to the ulcer. You can purchase the capsules at any health food store. Leave the ulcer open to the air as much as possible.

ALL WOUNDS AND ULCERS: Apply powdered sugar directly to the wound or ulcer. Change bandage each time you apply the powdered sugar. Sugar will help wounds to heal rapidly. This was used back in the Civil War and was said to have saved many a leg and arm.

TO PREVENT BED SORES: Allow the patient to lie on a fleecy pad. You can purchase these from a hospital if you can not find them at a store. Sheep wool is the best to use.

TREATING BED SORES: If the sore is open, pack the area with powdered sugar and cover with an airtight bandage. Change the bandage daily, morning and evening, washing the area with calendula liquid gently before putting fresh sugar and a bandage on the sore.

BED SORE TREATMENT: Put honey on a gauze pad and apply to the sore each night. Change the bandage the next morning after washing gently. Apply the honey bandage again. Should heal within 2 weeks.

BED SORES: Mix cornstarch and flower of sulfur. Dust the bed sores lightly to keep the sores free from infection.

RELIEVING THE PAIN OF BED SORES: After cleaning the sores carefully, break open a vitamin E capsule and apply directly to the sore. This relieves the pain and speeds healing.

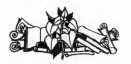

SPRAIN POULTICE: Bring to a boil 1/4 cup of vinegar. Add enough cayenne pepper to make a paste. Apply olive oil to the skin before applying this poultice. Spread the paste on a bandage and apply to the sprained area. Leave on for 2 hours. Rinse off any remaining pepper. Should relieve the pain and speed healing.

SPRAIN TREATMENT: Soak a piece of bread in hot apple cider vinegar and place on the affected area. Cover and allow to stay on the area at least 4 hours. Reduces swelling and relieves pain. If the area is too large to cover with the bread, dip a flannel cloth in the hot vinegar and wrap the area. Cover this with a plastic of some sort and leave on for 4 hours.

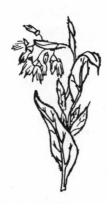

Comfrey (Symphytum officinale)

SPRAINS: Apply a poultice made from comfrey to relieve sprains and swellings. The Indians called this herb *knitbone* and used it extensively.

SPRAIN AND ACHING MUSCLES TREATMENT: Mix together 1/2 cup of water, 1/2 cup of linseed oil and 4 tablespoons witch hazel. Use as a massage.

SPRAIN POULTICE: Grate raw carrots and apply to the sprain. Cover and allow to stay on sprained area for 30 minutes.

PULLED MUSCLES: Soak a flannel cloth in buttermilk and warm the cloth in the oven. Apply to the area needed and cover to keep warm.

MENTHOL CREAM: Mix together 6 ounces of witch hazel, 4 teaspoons lanolin, and 6 teaspoons of menthol in a double boiler until creamy. Remove from fire and cool in the refrigerator. Use as a massage.

SWOLLEN JOINTS: Heat 1 cup of water and 1 cup of apple cider vinegar. Apply as a poultice to the affected joint. Cover to keep warm. Keep applying the vinegar and water mix for at least 30 minutes. Very soothing.

GOUT TREATMENT: Add 1 cup of cherry stems to 1 pint of water. Simmer for 30 minutes. Strain and add 1 pint of honey to the liquid. Take several tablespoons daily to prevent gout.

GOUT TREATMENT: Strawberry tea is good to use in treating gout. Place 4-5 leaves in a cup of boiling water and allow to steep 15 minutes. Strain and drink hot with honey.

GOUT TREATMENT: A diet of nothing but strawberries for 2 days is said to cure gout.

GOUT PREVENTION: Eating 3 fresh pears a day will help to stop attacks of gout.

GOUT TREATMENT: Mix equal amounts of sour cream and olive oil and apply to the joint affected. Apply flannel cloth to keep warm.

GOUT TREATMENT: Put 1 tablespoon of chopped blackcurrant leaf in 1 cup of water. Bring to a boil and reduce heat. Simmer for 10 minutes. Strain and drink 1/3 of the liquid 3 times daily.

GOUT TREATMENT: Dry some apple slices and save them to make a tea for treating gout. Put several of the slices in boiling water and steep for 15 minutes. Sweeten with honey and drink with each meal.

POULTICE FOR GOUT: Place the rind of a lemon on the affected joint and wrap up the joint to keep warm.

BURSITIS: Massage the affected area with warm olive oil on a daily basis. This might stop the return of bursitis, and it helps to relieve the pain.

BURSITIS RELIEF: Add 1 tablespoon of cayenne pepper to 1 cup of apple cider vinegar and bring to a boil. Simmer for 15 minutes. Dip a cloth in the liquid and apply to the affected area as a poultice. Rub the area with warm olive oil before applying the poultice.

BURSITIS TREATMENT: Grate 1 potato and add to a cup of water. Steep overnight. Strain the next morning and drink the liquid before breakfast. Should be done on a daily basis to prevent bursitis.

BURSITIS TREATMENT: Sea water has been reputed to cure chronic bursitis. Drink daily. Buy the sea water from a local health food store and drink one glass daily. *Caution:* DO NOT USE THIS RECIPE IF YOU HAVE HIGH BLOOD PRESSURE.

√ **PAIN:** Add several drops of lavender oil to your bath to relieve neuralgia (spasms of pain).

PAIN RELIEF: Grate a fresh horseradish root. Moisten with water and place in a small porous bag. Use as a poultice over the affected joint.

TREATING RHEUMATIC JOINTS: Grind black mustard seeds and add to an equal amount of solid vegetable shortening. Rub on the affected joint.

PAIN RELIEF FOR RHEUMATIC JOINTS OR ARTHRITIS: Put 2 cups of rosemary in 3 cups of brandy. Steep for 1 week. Strain and use the liquid as a poultice for the affected joints.

ARTHRITIS TREATMENT: Fill #00 capsules with ginger and take 2 daily. This will reduce pain and swelling after several months of treatment.

√ **BATH TREATMENT FOR ARTHRITIS:** Put several cups of sea salt in hot bath water and soak in the bath for at least 20 minutes every day.

√ **BATH TREATMENT FOR ARTHRITIS:** Put 1 cup of Epsom salts in your bath water (draw the bath as hot as you can stand it) and soak 20 minutes a day.

ARTHRITIS TREATMENT: Put 2 tablespoons of cod-liver oil in a glass of warm milk and drink twice daily. This will reduce inflammation of the joint tissue, thus reducing pain.

ARTHRITIS TREATMENT: Mix 1 cup each of buckthorn bark, cayenne pepper, alfalfa, comfrey, white yarrow, yucca root, parsley, and black cohosh root. Grind up thoroughly and fill some #00 capsules with the herbal mixture. The first week take 1 capsule daily; the second week, take 2 capsules daily; and during the third week take 3 capsules daily.

ARTHRITIS TREATMENT: Barley tea is an excellent way to treat arthritis. Make a tea by soaking 1 cup of unhulled barley in 2 quarts of boiling water for 3 hours. Strain and keep refrigerated. Drink 1 cup twice daily.

ARTHRITIS TREATMENT: Put 2 tablespoons of brewers yeast in a glass of milk or juice and drink every morning.

ARTHRITIS TREATMENT: Mix 1 tablespoon each of corn silk, broom flowers, skullcap, and boneset. Pour 1 cup boiling water over 1 tablespoon of herb mixture and steep 15 minutes. Strain and sweeten. Drink with meals.

ARTHRITIS TREATMENT: Add 1 teaspoon of fresh parsley to 1 cup of boiling water. Let steep 15 minutes. Strain and sweeten. Add 1/2 teaspoon of fresh ginger to the tea and drink hot. Drink every meal.

ARTHRITIS COCKTAIL: Mix well 1 ounce of honey, 14 ounces of water and 1 ounce apple cider vinegar. Drink once a day. You should be free of symptoms after using daily for 1 month.

RHEUMATOID ARTHRITIS: Put 2 tablespoons of alfalfa seeds in 2 cups of water. Bring to a fast boil. Remove from heat and steep for 30 minutes. Strain and add 2 cups of water. Add 1/2 cup of honey. Drink all four cups each day for 2 weeks. You should notice quite an improvement when the 2 weeks are up. Make the tea fresh daily.

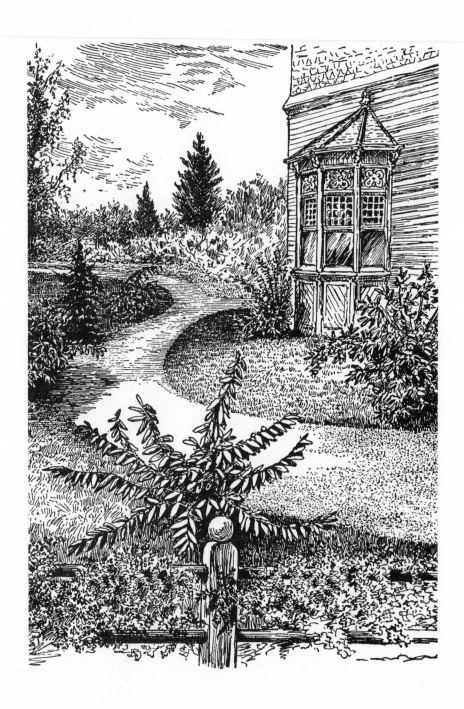

·11·

Preparations of Salves, Tinctures, Syrups and Capsules

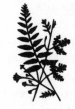

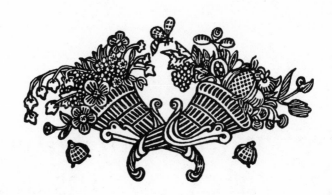

I n this chapter you can learn how to prepare your own salves, tinctures, syrups and capsules. I've also included many different recipes that use these different ways of preparing the herbs.

Preparing salves and liniments for future use is a good idea. It will save you time. If you prepare them in advance, you will have them on hand for emergencies or for everyday use. My daughter keeps a list of frequently used recipes taped inside the door of her herbal cabinet. Of course, there will always be recipes that you simply cannot prepare ahead of time, but their ingredients can be placed in tightly closed containers and clearly labeled. Always use sterile containers and be sure to clearly label each with the contents, use, and dosage.

It may take time to build up a nice supply of the kind of herbs needed for your remedies, but it is well worth the effort. If you are going to have a big supply of herbs, you must have containers in which to store them. I collect antique tin canisters and keep my dried herbs in them. Dark glass bottles are said to be the best kind of storage container, but I love my tins. I mainly use them for storing beeswax, capsules, and other miscellaneous things that I need to prepare herbal remedies. I place my canisters in a large cabinet that has glass doors. It holds a prominent place in my living room. It really does make a nice addition to the room and is very handy.

It is important to put a preservative in the recipes that you plan to store for indefinite periods of time. If honey is used in the recipe, that will be sufficient, as honey is a great preservative. If you are not using honey, adding the oil from several vitamin E capsules to your herbal mixtures is another way to preserve them. Gum benzoin is called for in some of the recipes. This is a preservative and you would not need to add any other preservatives if you were using it.

PREPARATION OF THE SALVES

Salves need a preservative because they are often used for cuts and wounds and as such need to be free from bacteria. A good preservative to use is tincture of benzoin, which you can purchase from your local drugstore. It is inexpensive and is necessary for the preparation of your salves. Choose stainless steel, glass, or earthenware when you are looking for bowls or containers in which to mix or store your herbal preparations. The containers you use to store the mixtures should be airtight and sterile.

It is helpful to know what the basic ingredients of a salve are. The ingredients used to make the salves are: the herbs you plan to use, an oil, beeswax, and the preservative. The best kind of oil to use is olive or sesame. Do not use the drying oils, such as soybean and linseed.

BASIC SALVE RECIPE: Begin by heating the oil just to boiling (in a stainless steel or glass pan). Add the herbs of your choice and simmer, covered, for about 3 hours. Instead of heating it up on the stove, you can prepare this mixture in the oven if you like. Just keep the temperature low and the container covered. If part of your herbal recipe includes barks or roots, place these in the oil first and simmer them for the first 1-1/2 hours before adding additional flowers or leaves. If using fresh herbs, always leave the lid off the container for the first 30 minutes in order to allow the water to evaporate from the herbs.

After the mixture is ready, strain and add the beeswax. (You will need about 1-1/2 ounces of beeswax for each pint of oil that you use.) Next, add 1/2 teaspoon of the tincture of benzoin for each pint of oil used. Mix well. To test for consistency, put a small amount of the salve in a tablespoon and place in the refrigerator. If the salve is not thick enough, add a little more beeswax. When the desired consistency is reached, pour into labeled jars.

The salve will keep for years. I place mine in small jars so that I have plenty to give family members and friends. These salves can also be used on your pets and animals.

Some of the following recipes will give the list of ingredients needed to prepare the remedy and then list each herb, with the reason why that particular herb was chosen. This should give you an understanding of the properties of the herbs and help you to make your own recipes. Carefully consider each of the herbs found in the recipes and look at the reasons behind their selection. Then you will know whether you would want to use that particular herb in that particular recipe. The following recipe and others like it in this chapter are designed to teach you to think more creatively about how herbal remedies are put together.

SALVE FOR ITCHING AND RASHES: Put 1 ounce of dried chickweed and 1 ounce of dried comfrey into 1 pint of olive oil and follow the instructions for the "Basic Salve Recipe." This salve is handy to have for treating diaper rash or for the itching caused by poison oak or poison ivy.

There are good reasons why chickweed works well for rashes. Chickweed has an active ingredient that is similar to something found in papaya. This ingredient helps to prevent the degeneration of cells. Papaya was also used by Native Americans as a meat tenderizer, and everyone knows that meat tenderizer is one of the best applications for bee and insect bites or stings. So, because the chickweed has similar properties, it acts in the same manner as the papaya.

Comfrey has many properties that make it useful for rashes. It has pain-killing properties and it is a great over-all healer. Allantoin is the substance responsible for most of the healing properties in comfrey. It allows skin tissue to heal much faster. The regenerative abilities of comfrey make it a great addition to salves. It is also very effective in destroying bacteria in wounds and cuts.

ALL PURPOSE SALVE: Mix together 1 ounce comfrey (aids in cell production, relieves pain), 1 ounce plantain leaves (also promotes healing), and 1 ounce calendula leaves (another great aid in preventing bacteria, healing. Studies have shown that calendula in water did slow the activity of some sarcomas (cancerous cells) in mice. The healing properties of calendula are a good addition to any salve. It is particularly appropriate for salves designed to treat sores or ulcers that have not responded very well to other methods or that have shown a resistance to healing.

PAIN RELIEVER SALVE: Mix together 1 ounce of chickweed (reduces inflammation and aids in healing), 1 ounce of wormwood (a great pain reliever), and 1 ounce of yarrow (an anti-bacterial agent that also helps to relieve pain).

The yarrow plant contains achillein and achilleic acid. These substances reduce the clotting time of blood, so they help stop any bleeding. Yarrow also has pain-killing and anti-inflammatory properties that are similar to aspirin.

Add the mixed herbs to 2 pints of olive oil and simmer 3 hours. Strain and add 3 ounces of beeswax and 1 teaspoon of tincture of benzoin. Test for consistency before pouring into wide mouth containers.

TAG ALDER SALVE: Add 1 ounce of tag alder bark to 1/2 pint of hot olive oil. Cover and simmer 3 hours. Add 3 ounces of beeswax and 1/4 teaspoon of tincture of benzoin to the strained mixture. Test for consistency and store in a labeled jar.

Tag alder's signature is the small corky warts on its bark, so this would indicate that it could be used for various skin disorders. Using the signatures of the herbs is another good way to tell what you could use in preparing the salves.

ALOE VERA SALVE: Pour 1 cup boiling water over 1 teaspoon of pekoe tea and 1 tablespoon of Irish moss. Allow to sit until cool. Add 3 tablespoons of aloe gel. Mix well and store in labeled jar.

Aloe contains a substance that is used to prepare the tincture of benzoin, so you would not need to add tincture of benzoin to preserve this recipe. Aloe is also a great healer and is very soothing for skin disorders. The Irish moss is a thickening agent, and becomes a jelly-like substance when added to a liquid. It also has healing and soothing agents in it. The pekoe tea contains tannin, which is a great healer. This salve can be used to heal burns, including sunburns.

MOISTURIZING OIL: Collect the flowers from mullein and place in an earthenware bowl. Macerate the flowers and cover with almond oil. Let stand for 1 week, covered. Strain and bottle. This is good for skin irritations, as well as being a great moisturizer.

ULCER OINTMENT: Good for leg ulcers. Melt 2 ounces of yellow beeswax and add to 8 ounces of honey. Mix well and apply to the ulcer twice daily. Change bandage with each application.

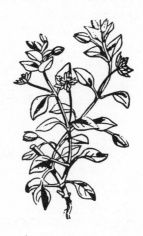

Chickweed (Stellaria media)

CHICKWEED SALVE: Add about 1 pound of chickweed to 1 pint of olive oil. Heat for 3 hours in an oven set at 150 degrees. Strain and add 1-1/2 ounces of melted beeswax to the mixture. Stir mixture while it is cooling, as it will thicken. Place in a wide mouth jar and label. Great for healing cuts, burns, and abrasions.

ALOE SALVE: Simmer 4 teaspoons of Irish moss in 1 pint of water for 10 minutes. Strain and add the juice and pulp of about 5 large aloe vera leaves. Use this salve for burns. It fights infection as well as speeding the healing of skin tissue.

AMARANTH SALVE: Place 1 ounce of dried amaranth flowers, leaves or roots in 1 pint of hot oil. Simmer, covered 2 hours. Remove from heat and strain. Add 1-1/2 ounces of beeswax and

1/2 teaspoon of tincture of benzoin to the mixture. Test for consistency and store in a tightly closed jar.

Amaranth has strong antiseptic and astringent properties. It can also help stop bleeding. This is a great salve to use for scrapes and cuts on children—particularly for knees and places that are constantly bumped, causing the sore to break open and start bleeding again. Stops the bleeding as well as keeps the sore free from bacteria.

POISON IVY SALVE: Add about 1 ounce each of dried cinquefoil, wild geranium, and powdered valerian root, dried, to 1 quart of water. Bring to a low boil and simmer until the mixture is halved. Strain and cool. Keep in the refrigerator and use as a compress as needed.

BALM OF GILEAD SALVE: Place 1 ounce of the buds in 1 pint of hot olive oil and allow to simmer, covered, 3 hours. Strain and add 1-1/2 ounces of beeswax and 1/2 teaspoon tincture of benzoin to the strained mixture. Test for consistency and place in sterile jar.

This is a good salve to use on burns, scratches, and swelling injuries. Also good for any skin eruptions. The signature of balm of Gilead is the resinous exudation covering the buds. It contains salicin, which is also found in aspirin. It has some of the same pain-killing and anti-inflammatory properties as aspirin.

GALL OINTMENT: This is a good ointment for soothing the skin after its been rubbed or chafed until irritated. I use it after I've worn a pair of shorts that rub me the wrong way. People who go horseback riding on a regular basis will also find it helpful.

Place 2 teaspoons each of lanolin and petroleum jelly in a pan. Cook on low heat until melted. Add 1 ounce of powdered galls. Stir until the mixture is cooled. Do not strain. Add a few drops of tincture of benzoin and store in a container.

GREEN ELDER OINTMENT: This is a good ointment to rub on the chest and back to relieve congestion. Put 1/2 pound of green elder leaves in 1 quart of vegetable oil. Heat in an oven for 3 hours at about 150 degrees. Strain and apply as chest and back rub. It's good to have this on hand during the winter season.

PREPARING TINCTURES

A tincture is nothing more than a highly concentrated liquid extract of herbs. A tincture can be applied externally or taken internally. The kind of herbs you choose to put in your tinctures depends upon what conditions you need to heal. For example, you would make a tincture of comfrey root to heal and clean sores, because comfrey has pain-killing properties and it also aids in cell rejuvenation. If you are choosing herbs to use in a tincture that will be taken orally, be careful to choose "safe" herbs, ones that you know you can safely ingest.

Here's how to make your own tincture: Add 4 ounces of the herb of your choice to 1 pint of alcohol. You can use vodka, rum, gin, or glycerin. The alcohol extracts the medicinal alkaloids and the volatile oils from the herbs. Allow the mixture to sit for about 2 weeks, shaking daily. Strain, pouring the liquid into a dark glass container which has been clearly labeled.

Tinctures can be used for many different illnesses. A tincture made from calendula flowers can be applied externally to cuts and scrapes, as well as taken orally for cramps and skin eruptions. When taken orally, dosage would be 5-15 drops for children and 10-25 drops for adults.

SEDATIVE TINCTURE: Place 1-1/2 ounces of chamomile and 1-1/2 teaspoons of powdered peppermint into 1/2 quart of vodka. Allow to steep for 2 weeks, shaking daily. Strain and bottle. Use as a sedative for adults. Dosage is 1/2 dropperful under the tongue, as needed.

VALERIAN ROOT TINCTURE: Although this tincture is a great sedative, I also use it to clean sores, cold sores, poison ivy rash, and a host of other skin ailments. It is wonderful for certain tension headaches and for sinus headaches. It is truly a great relaxant. Since it is a great muscle relaxant, it would be helpful to take orally for sore muscles or when suffering from back injury. Dosage for adults would be 1/2 dropperful every 4 hours or so for muscle spasms due to back pain. The smell is awful, so I place the liquid in #00 capsules and give the dosage that way. It goes down a lot easier.

Wild lettuce and skullcap would be good substitutes if valerian is not available. Both have a sedative effect. Just add 4 ounces of valerian (or the substitute herbs) to 1 pint of vodka or other alcohol and allow to sit for 2 weeks. Strain and bottle.

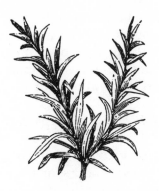

Rosemary (Rosemarinus officinalis)

ROSEMARY TINCTURE: This tincture is good to take internally to prevent colds or to fight infections. Because of the antibiotic nature of this tincture, it is also good to use to clean cuts and scrapes. It removes bacteria and prevents infections.

Add 4 ounces of rosemary needles to 1 pint of vodka and allow to sit for 2 weeks. Strain and use 1/2 dropperful every 2 hours for a couple of days. Then cut back to 2 times daily for about 2 weeks to treat infections and colds.

JUDE'S TINCTURE: I call this Jude's tincture because I don't know what else to call it. It works well and is very antibiotic in nature. It is great to use externally to clean cuts and scrapes. It will remove bacteria from cuts or wounds and prevent infections. I take it internally to prevent colds and to fight infections.

Add 1 ounce of macerated garlic, 1 ounce of yarrow, 1/4 ounce of echinacea root and 1 ounce of nasturtium leaves and flowers to 1 pint of vodka. Allow to sit for 2 weeks before straining. Shake daily. Strain and bottle.

The garlic is a natural antibiotic, the yarrow has aspirin-like substances and is a natural antiseptic. The nasturtium is a natural antiseptic and would help to clear mucus from the system. The echinacea root is a blood purifier and lymphatic cleanser as well as being an excellent antibiotic. Dosage would be 1/2 dropperful every couple of hours for 2-3 days. After a few days, take twice daily for 2 weeks to fight infections and colds.

YARROW TINCTURE: This is a good tincture to keep on hand to wash out wounds and sores. Add 1 cup fresh yarrow to 2 cups of vodka. Allow to sit for 2 weeks before straining and placing in a sterile bottle. The yarrow contains silacylates to stop pain. It also has antibiotic properties and will prevent infections.

ANTIBIOTIC TINCTURE: Add 2 cups garlic cloves, 2 cups of nasturtium leaves and flowers, and 2 cups of rosemary needles and stems to 1 quart of vodka. Let steep 2 weeks and strain. Dosage is 1 dropperful every 2 hours for several days. This is used to fight off an infection.

SWEET WOODRUFF TINCTURE: Fill a pint jar with sweet woodruff and cover the herb with vodka. Allow to sit in the sun for 3 weeks. Strain, bottle and label. Dosage is 1 dropperful every 4 hours, as a tonic for the liver and heart. Keep this treatment up for 1 week.

CALENDULA TINCTURE: Using oils to prepare tinctures is another way to make them. Many times a single herb is all that is necessary to use in preparing a home remedy. Calendula is one that serves many purposes and is handy to keep around. This is one that you would want to have in your herbal medicine chest.

Add 1 cup of calendula flower petals to 2 cups of olive oil. Allow to stand in a warm place for 2 weeks. Strain and add several drops of tincture of benzoin. Store in a sterile bottle. Use this to treat sores and chapped skin, to clean out wounds and cuts. Calendula helps stop bleeding so it could be used as a styptic. The tincture of benzoin keeps the herbal mixture bacteria-free and enables you to keep it for long periods of time. After you have started using your own tinctures, it will surprise you how often you will turn to them when needed.

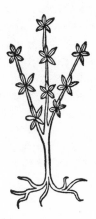

Sweet Woodruff (Galium odoratum)

SWEET WOODRUFF OINTMENT: Fill a pint jar with dried sweet woodruff and pour olive oil over the herb to fill the jar. Place in the sun for 2 weeks and strain. Add several drops of tincture of benzoin to the mixture before placing it in a labeled bottle. This can be applied to any cut, scrape or wound. Sweet woodruff has long been used to aid in the healing of wounds. It has also been used for centuries as a perfume base. This recipe could be applied to the skin as a scent, as well as for medicinal purposes.

The scent of sweet woodruff gets stronger the longer it dries. The herb's vanilla scent comes from an organic compound called coumarin. Coumarin is used in making perfumes and was the first natural scent to be synthesized from coal-tar products.

TINCTURE FOR TEENAGERS: Place 1/2 cup chopped onion in 1 cup of olive oil and allow to steep for 2 weeks. Strain and bottle. Use on pimples to help dry them up. Allow the liquid to stay on the spots for 15 minutes before rinsing off.

EARACHE TINCTURE: Fill a small jar with mullein flowers and cover with olive oil. Allow to stand in the sun for 1 week, shaking daily. Strain and place in sterile jar. Apply 3-4 drops to affected ear as needed and cover with a warm cloth.

✓ **CLOVE OIL:** Clove oil is great to use for toothaches. You can make your own by mixing together equal amounts of whole cloves and vegetable oil and allowing it to sit for several weeks. I use this oil as an addition to my potpourri pot when simmering scented water. Cinnamon oil can be made the same way. Simply pour the oil over cinnamon sticks and allow to sit for several weeks. Not only does this save you money, but these oils are handy to have around.

PREPARING LINIMENTS AND RUBS
FOR SPRAINS AND ARTHRITIC CONDITIONS

One of the best rubs I know is camphorated oil. Because it is no longer sold commercially, it may be necessary to make your own. You can purchase some small, 1 ounce camphor blocks from your local druggist. If it is not in stock, ask your druggist to order it for you, or to please stock it for you. Most druggists are very pleasant and helpful if you tell them why you need a certain product.

The camphorated oil is cheap to make and very handy to have around. It makes a good chest rub for chest colds as well being good for arthritic conditions. Shave the block of camphor in an earthenware or glass bowl, and add 1 ounce of menthol crystals. This too can be purchased at your local drug store. When you add the menthol crystals, the menthol and camphor will melt into a liquid. Add the resulting liquid to 1 pint of heavy mineral oil, or if not available, add to 1 pint of olive oil. Shake well and it is ready to use. This really works well to treat arthritis and rheumatism, as well as for strained or pulled muscles. I use it for chest congestion during colds to ease breathing.

Caution: DO NOT DRINK THIS LIQUID, it is for external use only. Rub on the affected areas for treatment of arthritis. If used to treat a chest ailment, rub on and cover the area with several thicknesses of flannel to hold in the heat.

LINIMENT FOR COLDS AND CHEST TIGHTNESS: Add 1 cup of finely chopped garlic to 1 cup of boiling lard. Reduce heat to simmer and cook for 2 hours. Remove from heat and strain the garlic from the oil. Place in a container with a tight-fitting lid.

LINIMENT FOR SPRAINS AND SORE JOINTS: Mix 2 table-spoons of freshly grated horseradish with 1 cup of vegetable oil. Bring to a boil and lower heat. Simmer for 10 minutes. Strain and store in labeled bottles.

LINIMENT FOR SPRAINS AND SORE JOINTS: Mix together 1 cup of turpentine and 2 cups of vegetable oil. Use as a massage oil.

LINIMENT FOR SORE MUSCLES: Mix together 1/4 cup each of olive oil and spirits of camphor. Use to massage sore muscles.

PULLED LIGAMENTS: Place a large onion in the blender and blend until completely pulverized. Add 1 cup of olive oil and blend until smooth. Spread on a clean cloth and use as a poultice for pulled muscles. Cover to keep warm. This is good to keep on hand if you have kids who play football.

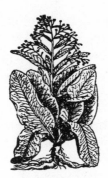

Horseradish (Cochlearia armoracia)

ARTHRITIS LINIMENT: Put 1 cup each of melted paraffin and grated horseradish in the blender. Blend until liquefied. Rub the affected joint with the mixture and wrap loosely with a flannel cloth. Leave on overnight. Rinse off the next morning. Repeat until swelling is gone. The horseradish liniment should be stored in a tightly closed container at room temperature.

SKIN OINTMENT: Use this for a multitude of skin disorders. Mix 2 cups of olive or vegetable oil with 2 cups of calendula petals and leaves. Place pan in an oven at low heat (about 150 degrees) and heat for several hours. Strain well and add 1/4 teaspoon of tincture of benzoin. Pour into a sterile bottle.

RHEUMATIC PAIN OINTMENT: Place 1/2 cup of rosemary leaves and 1/2 teaspoon oil of cloves in 1 cup of vegetable oil. Simmer gently for 20 minutes. Strain well and bottle. Make a poultice and use as often as necessary for rheumatic pain.

ARTHRITIS LINIMENT: Rub this liniment in every morning if needed. Can be left on the skin until the next day. Mix 1/2 cup each of salt and dry mustard. Add enough melted paraffin to make a paste. Rub on the affected area. Helps to relieve swelling and pain.

ARTHRITIS TREATMENT: Mix together 1/2 cup each of apple cider vinegar, turpentine, and either olive or vegetable oil. Rub on the affected joints each night before bed.

WORMWOOD LINIMENT: To 1 gallon of white vinegar, add 4 ounces wormwood herb and seed. Let sit for 2 weeks. Strain, bottle and label. When the time comes to use this remedy, beat 4 egg whites. Slowly add 1 quart of the wormwood mixture and 4 ounces of pure turpentine. Keep tightly capped. Shake well before using. Saturate bandages and wrap around the legs when needed. This is good to use for arthritis and stiffness.

This recipe came from Ella Birzneck, who was President of Dominion Herbal College until her death in 1989. Originally, the liniment was used for horses to treat rheumatism, stiff joints, and swollen legs for horses. A friend of Mrs. Birzneck's used it on his horse and it worked so well that he tried it on his own knees. It worked. I'm sorry I did not get to meet Mrs. Birzneck before her death. She sounded like a very interesting lady.

ARTHRITIS, RHEUMATISM, AND STIFF JOINTS: Mix together 2 ounces mullein herb, 1 teaspoon of cayenne pepper, and 1/2 ounce lobelia. Add to 2 quarts of cider vinegar. Simmer for 30 minutes. Strain. To use, reheat and dip cloth into mixture and use as a compress over the affected areas.

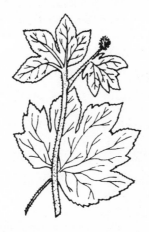

Goldenseal (Hydrastis canadensis)

LINIMENT FOR ACHING BODY: Add 2 ounces of powdered goldenseal to 1 quart of rubbing alcohol. Let sit for 2 weeks, shaking daily. Use as a massage for aching muscles.

ARTHRITIS LINIMENT: Add 1-1/2 tablespoons of bruised mustard seeds and 1/4 cup of cayenne pepper to 1 pint of whiskey. Simmer for about 10 minutes and strain. Dip cloth in the liquid while hot and apply to affected joint. Bottle and reuse by heating the liquid each time. Relieves pain fast. *Caution:* Apply warm olive oil to the area before applying the poultice.

WINTERGREEN RUB: Add 1 dram of wintergreen to 1 pint of witch hazel. Bottle and label. Use as a massage for sprains and sore muscles.

ARTHRITIS TREATMENT: Here's a recipe that's included just for curiosity's sake. When applied to the affected joint, stinging nettle is reputed to relieve pain within several hours. I add this just as a curiosity. I don't believe I would use this as it could be very uncomfortable.

ARTHRITIS TREATMENT: Mix 1 quart of apple cider vinegar to 1 quart of hot water. Dip a cloth into the hot vinegar water and apply as a compress to the affected area. Put a heating pad over the compress and keep on for 30 minutes.

MUSCLE PAIN: Mix 1 teaspoon cayenne pepper with a small bottle of olive oil. Massage aching muscles as often as necessary to relieve pain.

SPRAINS: Bruise a couple of handfuls of sage leaves. Use dried sage if fresh is not available. Put the sage in 1/2 pint of vinegar and boil for 5 minutes. Dip a cloth in the boiling-hot vinegar and herb mixture and wring it out. Apply it to the sprain. Make sure the cloth is as hot as you can stand it.

LINIMENT: Add 1 tablespoon each of cayenne pepper, wormwood, and tansy flowers to 8 ounces of cider vinegar. Warm gently for 1 hour. Cool, strain, and add 1/2 ounce spirits of camphor and 8 ounces of turpentine to the herbal vinegar. After rubbing the affected area with the liniment, cover with a flannel cloth to keep warm. This is good for just about any stiffness, arthritis, rheumatism or sore muscles.

GALL OINTMENT: Simmer 1 ounce of plantain leaves and 1 ounce ground oak galls in 4 ounces of solid vegetable shortening for 30 minutes. Strain, then cool. Add 1-1/2 teaspoons tincture of benzoin, stirring well. Rub on the affected area.

RASH SALVE: Add 16 ounces of fresh chickweed, 8 ounces comfrey, 8 ounces calendula, 8 ounces plantain leaves and 2 ounces of beeswax to 32 ounces of olive oil. Simmer several hours. Strain and add 1 teaspoon of gum benzoin. Let cool in the refrigerator, testing for consistency. If too thin, reheat and add more beeswax. This is very good for itching caused by poison ivy, diaper rash, heat rash, or just about any kind of rash. The gum benzoin will preserve this mixture. Add vitamin E oil if that is not handy.

MARSH MALLOW OINTMENT: Bruise 1/2 pound each of marsh mallow leaves and fresh elder flowers. Add to 1/2 pound of melted vegetable shortening along with 1 ounce of melted beeswax. Simmer for 30 minutes. Strain and cool. Stir the mixture while it is cooling. Label and store. This makes a good all-around salve. Good for skin ulcers, as well as for scrapes and cuts on children.

ALL PURPOSE HEALING SALVE: Mix together 2 ounces of comfrey leaves, 1 ounce of plantain leaves, 1 ounce of yarrow, 1 ounce of calendula, 1 ounce wormwood leaves, 1 ounce chickweed leaves and 1-1/2 ounces of beeswax. Simmer for several hours. Strain and add 1 teaspoon gum benzoin. Cool and test for consistency. Put in sterile jar. Label and use on any cut, scrape or rash.

BURN OINTMENT: Squeeze 10 vitamin E capsules in 1/4 cup of extra virgin olive oil. Apply to the burn frequently. Prevents scar tissue from forming.

CANKER AND COLD SORE OINTMENT: Dry and grind the rind from a pomegranate. Put 2 tablespoons of the dried pomegranate in 1-1/2 cups of water. Bring to a boil and reduce heat to a simmer. Simmer until the liquid is reduced by half. Strain and store in the refrigerator. Use as a rinse for canker sores and apply as a wash for the cold sores.

MULLEIN OINTMENT: This is used to treat frostbite, hemorrhoids, chapped skin, and earaches. This can also be used to remove warts, if used as a poultice.

Steep the flowers of mullein in olive oil for 1 month. Strain well and store in tightly closed bottle. Label the bottle, listing the ingredients and the disorders it can treat.

OINTMENT FOR WOUNDS: St. John's wort *(hypericum perforatum)* is really a wonderful tincture to keep around. It kills harmful bacteria as well as pain. To make the tincture to use on wounds (especially dirty wounds), put 1 ounce of St. John's wort in 1 pint of boiling water. Cover and steep for 30 minutes. Strain well and add 1 cup of sugar. Use this to clean wounds. Change the bandage frequently and wash the wound each time with the tincture.

Here's another variation: Put 1 ounce of the herb in 1 pint of witch hazel and allow to steep for 2 weeks before straining. This makes a good wash for wounds. Be sure to label all bottles with the ingredients and their use.

PREPARATION OF DECOCTIONS AND SYRUPS

As you become more experienced in working with the herbs, you will find the confidence to create your own recipes. To help you do that, I am giving you more recipes that include explanations of why each herb is included. You might also want to refer to the list of categories given toward the end of chapter one. The categories listed are: stimulants, diuretics, expectorants, astringents, nervines and tonics. Herbs from one category can be substituted for another from the same category. Of course, not all of the herbs in each of these categories are equal to each other as far as their potency and their secondary effects, so a little research will help you select the appropriate herbs from the categories. Otherwise, you can simply follow the recipes outlined in this book. Just remember to use the herbs responsibly. When in doubt, consult your health care expert.

For the recipes in this section, the herbs should be dried. When preparing the cough syrups, the dried herbal mixtures are generally decocted (boiled). The mixture is then strained. Then the honey is added and the mixture is allowed to simmer an additional 30 minutes. Add the flavoring after the mixture has cooled. (Wild cherry oil is a great flavor addition.)

There are certain types of herbs that are generally included when preparing cough syrups. They are as follows:

1. Stimulants or activators: A stimulant is an agent that temporarily increases functional activity. For example, a diuretic increases the secretion of urine. If a diuretic is desired, these herbs would be good choices: parsley, watercress, and asparagus leaves or roots. If a diaphoretic is wanted, you could use boneset, yarrow, peppermint or verbena. A diaphoretic is an agent or sudorific that increases perspiration.

2. Aromatics: Aromatics have a pleasant smell. Some good examples are mints, fennel, catnip, sassafras bark, and marjoram.

3. Demulcents: Here are some examples: mallow, hollyhocks, Irish moss, mullein, slippery elm, honey, and balm of Gilead. A demulcent is an agent that soothes or softens. It usually aids the mucous membranes.

BASIC COUGH SYRUP RECIPE: Mix together these dried herbs: 1/2 teaspoon thyme, 1 teaspoon boneset, 1 teaspoon lobelia, 1 teaspoon elecampane, 2 teaspoons Irish moss, 1 teaspoon coltsfoot, 1 teaspoon slippery elm, 1 teaspoon wild cherry bark, 1 teaspoon yarrow, 1 tablespoon balm of Gilead, 1 tablespoon mullein, and 1 tablespoon peppermint.

Add the dried herbal mixture to 1 quart of water and boil until the mixture is halved. Strain well and add 1 pint of honey. Simmer an additional 30 minutes. Cool and add flavoring if desired.

Now, let's look at the ingredients more closely and see why we are using these particular herbs in this cough syrup.

Thyme has antispasmodic properties. This makes it effective to use for coughs and colds. The tendency of the herb to branch out as it grows is the signature of the plant. In this way, it relates to the "branches" found in the bronchial, alimentary and urinary systems.

Lobelia is an expectorant, so it is good to use in cough syrups. It is also called asthma weed. It is prominent in remedies for treatment of asthma and bronchial disorders. The signature is the swollen seed capsules. They swell when it is time to collect them. The swollen seeds are indicators for all swellings and sprains, or for swollen conditions related to wet colds or chest ailments. Use the herb externally in a hot compress for swelling injuries or for sprains.

Elecampane is used because of its soothing properties. It was one of the main ingredients in a cough syrup recipe that comes to us from the Native American tradition. Here is the recipe: Make a cough syrup by combining 1/2 pound each of elecampane root, spikenard root, and comfrey root. Mash the roots well and add them to a gallon of water. Boil the liquid until it is reduced by half and add 1/2 pint each of brandy and honey. Simmer an additional 30 minutes. The dose would be 1 teaspoon every hour (or as needed).

Elecampane's yellow flowers are one of the plant's signatures. They signify that the herb is useful to the urinary system. In this case, elecampane helps induce urination, which is very useful when you have a cold. It helps you flush the toxins out of your body's system.

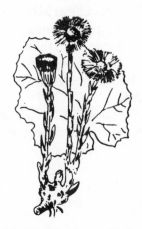

Coltsfoot (Tussilago farfara)

Coltsfoot is also called coughwort. The ancient Romans called it *tussilago*, which means cough plant. The principle active ingredient in coltsfoot is a throat-soothing mucilage. At one time coltsfoot was used as a tobacco for asthmatics. But studies have shown that the mucilage is destroyed by burning and so coltsfoot really has no therapeutic value as a tobacco. The herb's signature is that when its leaves are pressed together, they stay together. This led early herbalists to believe that the herb's active substance would stick to the toxins in the body. After that substance attaches itself to the toxins, the toxins can then be removed through the urinary tract. This is also true of horehound and sage. Both can be substituted for coltsfoot. The flowers of coltsfoot are yellow; this signifies that the herb is also diuretic in nature.

Boneset has been used to improve the condition of the mucous membranes of the alimentary and bronchial systems, the bowels and the liver. It was also used by Native Americans as a diaphoretic, based on the belief that sweating out the toxins will help you heal. It grows in swamps or along the banks of rivers and streams, so could be used for colds, influenza or other "wet"diseases.

It's history is interesting. It was used by early herbalists to set bones. The leaves were softened with water, wrapped around the injured area, and then bandaged tightly, often with a splint. This was a very primitive way of dealing with broken bones and should

NOT be used today. See your doctor for any bone break. There can be serious complications from broken bones, so don't fool around—get proper medical attention.

The flowers are white, so I would consider it a good tonic to take as a blood purifier during times of illness.

Balm of Gilead is actually the poplar tree buds, gathered in very late winter or early spring. The buds are considered to be a stimulating expectorant for bronchial disorders. Balm of Gilead has a soothing effect upon the throat so would be great to add to cough syrups, as it has a numbing substance that stops pain. When preparing an ointment, the buds are sometimes simmered in lard. When preparing a tincture to heal skin eruptions, bruises, cuts or scrapes, they are placed in alcohol.

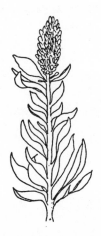

Mullein (Verbascum thapus)

Mullein is also called lungwort. It is a demulcent and an emollient. It has pain-relieving properties. It also serves as an antibiotic because it can inhibit certain types of bacteria. The signature of mullein is the yellow flowers, signifying that it can be used as a diuretic; the woolly hairs on the leaves indicate a tickling sensation to the throat, therefore it would be used in treatment of the bronchial system. Horehound can be substituted for mullein, although I prefer mullein.

Irish moss is an emollient that stops coughs due to colds. Not only is it good to use for bronchial disorders, but it is also used for kidney or bowel complaints. The signature is its resemblance to the human bronchial system and the fact that when placed in hot water, the dried plant will yield a thick mucilaginous jelly.

Peppermint has the distinct ability to eliminate hardening mucus from the alimentary and bronchial systems and to prevent further discomforts caused by mucus. Used with boneset and sage, it is considered a diaphoretic and can be used in a tea to treat colds. Its signature is that it grows in wet or mucky soils, thus it can be used for wet diseases of the bronchial system.

Slippery elm is an emollient and a demulcent. The dried inner bark of the tree is the part used to prepare medicinal remedies. It is a great expectorant and helps to dispel phlegm. The signature is the bland mucilaginous substance that can be found by chewing the bark.

Wild cherry bark is astringent in nature. The gum, dissolved in a suitable base, is used as a pectoral sedative in cough syrup preparations. The bark can be used externally for cuts and sores as a decoction, as well as for bronchial disorders.

Yarrow can be added to the cough syrup because of it's aspirin-like substances as well as its antibiotic properties. It will soothe the pain while the antibiotic properties fight the infection.

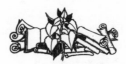

EASY ELECAMPANE COUGH SYRUP: Pour 1 cup water over 1 cup elecampane root and add 1 cup of honey. Bring to a quick boil, reduce heat to simmer. Simmer until the root is soft. Strain and take as needed for coughs.

ONION COUGH SYRUP: Every one knows the astringent properties of onions. There's nothing better to treat a cough. Chop 1 pound of onions very fine. Add to 2 pints of water. Add 1 pound of brown sugar and 3 ounces of honey. Simmer for 4 hours, covered. Strain the onions from the liquid and place in labeled bottle. Take 1 tablespoon as needed for coughs.

MAKING COUGH DROPS

You can make your own cough drops by using the herb of your choice. Choose any of the herbs that are soothing, cooling, and astringent—or any that are used in preparing the cough syrups. To really soothe the throat, use balm of Gilead along with an aromatic herb.

You can even flavor your cough drops with herbs. Lemon flavor can be made by using lemon balm, lemon thyme, or lemon verbena. Licorice mint makes an excellent-tasting cough drop, as it has a light licorice flavor. Color the drops using food coloring if desired. Using horehound as an example, try this recipe substituting an herb of your choice.

HOREHOUND COUGH DROPS: Simmer 1 cup of horehound leaves and 1 tablespoon of balm of Gilead in 1 pint of water for about 15 minutes. Strain and add 2 cups of sugar. Boil until the mixture spins a thread as it comes off of the spoon. Drop by the teaspoonful into cold water to form the cough drops. Remove the cough drops from the water immediately. You can roll the cough drops in powdered sugar after draining off the water. This will keep them from sticking to each other. Place in a tightly sealed container.

Experiment with different herbs to make the cough syrups or drops. You will soon find a recipe that suits you. As you prepare the mixtures, you will become more familiar with the properties of the herbs. The only way to learn anything is the hands-on approach. Don't just talk the talk. Walk the walk and become acquainted with the herbs through practical use.

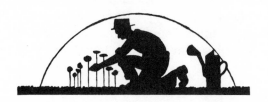

TREATMENT FOR HEADACHES AND BACKACHES

Mix together 1 tablespoon each of dried yarrow, boneset, and skullcap. Add the mixture to 1 pint of water and simmer 30 minutes, covered. Strain and add 1 tablespoon of the liquid to 1 cup of hot water. Add 1 teaspoon of flavored psyllium. Sweeten with 1 tablespoon of dark corn syrup if desired.

Yarrow is used in this recipe because it is a wonderful tonic for the whole body. The herb grows in all of the northern temperate countries and in any type of soil. The whole plant is covered with grayish silky hairs and the leaves have many divisions, thus many different uses. The root system's branching tendencies suggests that it has blood-cleansing properties. It has many blood-fortifying minerals, such as iron, calcium, sulfur and potassium. It also has pain-killing properties, which is another reason we use it in this recipe.

Boneset is generally used with other laxative herbs. It is a wonderful tonic, as it has a cleansing effect upon all the organs. It is also a muscle relaxant and can be used in treating muscular rheumatism. It has been considered a near cure-all for many centuries.

Skullcap's signature is the bell-shaped lid of the calyx. The calyx is a cap or helmet-shaped protuberance; it looks like a little dish for the head. It is a superior nervine and tonic. It is a good relaxant and is useful for sleeplessness, headaches and all nervous disorders.

Psyllium's signature is the amount of mucilage in the seeds. It is used extensively in laxative preparations. It helps to clean the intestinal tract and helps with lower back pain that is related to constipation or bowel problems.

PREPARING CAPSULES

Herbal remedies may be taken in capsule form as well as by teas or tinctures. Often, capsules are more convenient to take during the day while we are at work, or while away from home for an extended length of time. There are many reasons that you would want to take capsules instead of a tea or tincture. If the treatment you are seeking is long term, such as for high blood pressure, then you would definitely want to try the capsules.

You can purchase the empty gelatin capsules at your local health food store or druggist's. There are many different sizes of capsules, but you probably would use the #00 capsules the most. To fill the capsules, simply take them apart and fill the largest end of the capsules, replacing the top to close it. The leafy herbs can be powdered in your food processor if necessary, but the root herbs must be purchased in powdered form.

The dosage would be the same as if you were taking an infusion, which is a tea remedy. If the infusion calls for 3 cups a day, then you would take 1 capsule three times a day with water.

We will start with the blood pressure capsules. If you are already on a medication or need to take a medication to control your blood pressure, *please do not substitute these capsules for your regularly prescribed medication.*

BLOOD PRESSURE CAPSULES: Mix together in the blender or food processor 1 tablespoon of each of the following dried herbs: stinging nettle, spearmint, elder flowers, powdered valerian root, lobelia, chamomile, and yarrow.

This makes enough capsules to last about 1-1/2 months if taken on a daily basis. The reasons for using these herbs in this recipe are listed in the following paragraphs.

Stinging nettle has been used extensively as a weight reduction herb. It helps to dispel toxins and water from the body. The signature of the plant is the stinging hair that covers the entire herb. Other uses include treating any stitching pain, such as in arthritis, or in any pain that causes that "pins and needles" feeling. It has also been used as a remedy to stimulate hair growth.

Spearmint prefers to grow in moist ground and this is the signature of the plant. It is used as a diuretic in this recipe. Treatments for high blood pressure generally remove excess water from the system and this is why you need to use diuretics. Spearmint can be used in any recipe that is used to treat inflammatory problems of the bladder and kidneys. It is also a stimulant, and can be used in recipes calling for a stimulant.

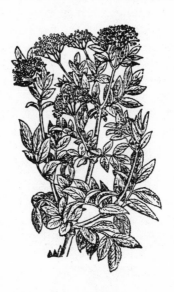

Elder (Sambucas nigra)

Elder is also called boretree. It is found in low, moist ground and has the yellowish-gray bark that is part of its signature. The fresh stems can be made fully hollow by pushing out the soft pith. This hollowing represents the herb's healing properties, as it effectively helps to push out the mucous deposits from the bronchial tubes. Because of this, it is a natural choice for remedies designed to treat colds, coughs, and chest complaints.

The freshly dried leaves and flowers can be used to prepare ointments and creams to help the healing of skin disorders and itching. An infusion of the flowers in vinegar is a good, healing ointment to keep on hand for skin problems. It is in this recipe because it is also a diuretic and helps to clear the body of toxins.

Valerian's fine, delicate root system is thought to resemble the human brain structure. It has an outstanding influence on the cerebospinal system and is an easily tolerated calmative. It also acts as a stimulant and diuretic for the kidneys, and so you could use it to treat kidney problems.

Lobelia affects the central nervous system and is a good muscle relaxant. When used with care, this can be a good treatment for high blood pressure because it depresses the central nervous system and lowers the blood pressure. *Caution:* Do not use more than the recipe calls for, as it can be harmful if used in too large of a dose, lowering the blood pressure too drastically and too fast.

Chamomile's signature is the head-shaped flowers. It is a calmative and sedative, which is why it was chosen for this recipe. One of the ways to lower the blood pressure is to keep the patient as calm as possible. *Caution:* Do not use this herb if you suffer from ragweed allergies, as chamomile is a member of the ragweed family. Use one of the other herbs that have sedative properties, such as hops, violets, or any of the nervines listed in chapter one.

Yarrow is used because it contains potassium. It is a good blood cleanser and it fortifies the blood with necessary minerals. Anyone taking any type of blood pressure treatment should take a potassium supplement, as the diuretics flush the potassium from the body. It needs to be replaced so the heart is not affected adversely.

CIRCULATION PROBLEMS

High cholesterol is the main reason that we have poor circulation, along with other factors such as poor diet and pollution. When you have one health problem, there are generally three or four other conditions involved. When the circulation is poor, there are almost always other related problems such as varicose veins, poor memory, hemorrhoids, and forgetfulness.

MEMORY RETENTION RECIPE: Try this recipe for memory retention caused by poor circulation. Take the herbal capsules along with a multiple vitamin B complex tablet.

Mix together in the food processor 1 tablespoon each of the following herbs: butcher's broom, lecithin, apple pectin, and cayenne pepper. Place in #00 capsules. Take 2 capsules morning and evening. For the first month, take a vitamin B complex tablet with the morning capsule. Thereafter, take 2 capsules daily and continue taking 1 tablet of the B complex vitamins daily.

The herbs used in this recipe are used for the following reasons:

Butcher's broom has been used for circulation problems for over two thousand years. It is also used to prevent blood clots after surgery.

Lecithin dissolves fatty deposits in the circulatory systems by attaching itself to the deposits. Since it is water soluble, it flushes the deposits from the system.

Apple pectin has magnetic properties that attract ions of metal in the blood such as lead, arsenic, and other pollutants. These are then flushed from the system. Pectin also regulates the bowels and is effective in lowering cholesterol levels in the blood.

Cayenne pepper kills bacteria in the blood and carries nutrients to the place they are needed faster than any other natural agent. Cayenne is used for many kinds of treatment. It can lower blood pressure as well as dissolve cholesterol deposits. It is also helpful for the heart and stomach.

LUNG CONGESTION AND SINUS TREATMENT

Using herbs for healing is important. When you take herbs, you allow nutrients to enter the body's system and that sometimes reduces the symptoms of some diseases. Herbs nourish, detoxify and stimulate the system.

The stimulating herbs help to increase the production of enzymes and hormones. They can stimulate the kidneys, helping them to remove harmful toxins from the body. Some of the herbs attract the toxins to them and then the toxins are passed through the system and out of the body. Many herbs will kill invading organisms and bacteria.

When congestion is present, no matter what the cause, the body produces mucus and phlegm to protect sensitive mucus membranes. This recipe contains herbs that will break up the congestion and pull it from the lungs and sinus cavity. Dosage would be 2 capsules every 2 hours for 3 days and then 2 capsules daily until symptoms are relieved.

Mix together in a blender or food processor 1 tablespoon each of the following herbs: 1 tablespoon fenugreek, 1 tablespoon slippery elm, 1 tablespoon thyme, and 1 tablespoon comfrey. Place in capsules and refer to the dosage suggestions.

Here are the reasons we are using these herbs:

Fenugreek is a germicidal for the lungs. It will act as a disinfectant and help to reduce inflammation.

Slippery elm will cause the loosened phlegm and mucus to ball up, which helps it move more easily out of the respiratory system. It also has healing and soothing properties to benefit the lungs.

Thyme is used mainly for its antiseptic properties, but it also has great expectorant properties. An expectorant is used to discharge the mucus from the body.

Comfrey root has been used since ancient times for congestion problems. It reduces inflammation and it breaks up congestion in the lungs.

FLU CAPSULES: This is a good capsule to take to lessen the length and severity of colds and flu. Mix together in the blender 1 tablespoon each of yarrow, elder flowers, boneset, verbena, peppermint, powdered valerian root, and horehound.

Place the herbal mixture in capsules and take 2 capsules every 3-4 hours until symptoms are relieved.

Yarrow is added because it contains salicylic acid derivatives, which do lessen the discomforts of the symptoms. Salicylic acid is in aspirin so it would reduce fever and fight pain or discomfort. Also, it contains azulene and other compounds that fight inflammations and infections. Yarrow is a great antiseptic.

Elder flowers are used in this recipe because the flowers stimulate secretion of the sweat glands. When sweating increases, fever tends to come down.

Boneset is used because it is a muscle relaxant, and a diaphoretic. It acts as a tonic for the whole body. It has a great cleansing effect on most of the body's organs.

Verbena is used because it settles the stomach and acts as a tonic for the stomach and intestines. Verbena has some sedative properties and will help to reduce fever.

Peppermint is used in this recipe to reduce nausea and promote digestion.

Valerian is a well known sedative. It can be used as a relaxant so that you get the rest you need during recovery from the flu. It also acts as a stimulant to the kidneys to rid the body of toxins.

Horehound is added because of its well known ability to remove mucus from the bronchial system. The signature is that the leaves do stick together when pressed. This would indicate that the herb has compounds that would stick to the toxins and remove them from the system.

CHANGE OF LIFE REMEDY

Because menopausal symptoms are the result of the depletion of estrogen hormones, you need to make a recipe that will nourish both the adrenal glands and the ovaries. The adrenal glands carry on the production of this hormone when the ovaries are missing.

A recipe to deal with menopausal symptoms should also include herbs that have estrogen-like properties. Wild yam root, black cohosh root, and licorice root are examples of this. We are not trying to replace the missing estrogen. We are teaching the body to replace the missing hormones; we are teaching the body to make it's own substitute.

This recipe uses the roots of the herbs. Purchase all of the herbal roots in powdered form so you can use them in the capsules. Mix together 1 tablespoon each of black cohosh, wild yam root, chamomile, licorice root, motherwort, skullcap, and valerian.

Mix together in food processor and place in capsules. Take 2 capsules three times daily until symptoms abate. Then take 2 capsules daily.

The following list of the herbs explains why they were used in this recipe.

Valerian is again used because it is a great sedative and helps to calm the whole system.

Black cohosh contains estrogen-like properties and is a muscle relaxant. It soothes nerves and general restlessness.

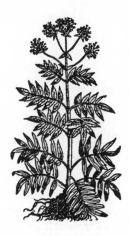

Valerian (Valerian officinalis)

Chamomile is used because it acts as a sedative and does have properties that will ease cramps and other gastrointestinal disorders.

Motherwort strengthens the nerve system and is a tonic for the whole body. It helps those who are prone to headaches and helps relieve menstrual discomforts.

Wild yam is reported to contain an estrogen-like molecule (diosgenin). When this molecule enters the body, it is treated and reacted to as an estrogen molecule by the body. This is why it is necessary to take a daily dose after you have reached menopause.

Licorice root also has estrogen-like properties and is included for that reason. It also nourishes the adrenal glands.

Skullcap is included because it is a great nervine and helps with sleep disorders and headaches.

This recipe is also good to take for the nervous disorders that you may suffer from during "change of life." Remember to purchase all of the herbs in a powdered form.

CALCIUM SUPPLEMENT: If you are in the menopausal years and are not now taking calcium, it is a good idea to start taking a calcium supplement on a regular basis. This builds bone mass as well as correcting fluid balance in the body. The calcium can be taken through the following herbs if desired: shepherd's purse, plantain, chamomile, coltsfoot, and sorrel.

ENERGY TONIC PILLS: Try this for extra energy during menopause or any other time. Mix 1 cup each of cayenne pepper, ginseng, and gotu kola. Fill #00 capsules. Take 2 capsules 3 times daily for 1 month. Stop for 2 weeks and begin taking again for another 4 weeks.

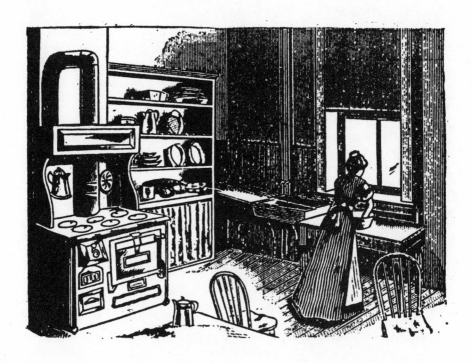

·12·

Pet Care and Garden Tips

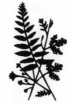

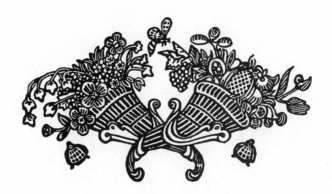

M any people have pets and many more already have the pleasure of keeping a garden. In this chapter, we will cover some recipes for pet care and also a few garden hints.

PET CARE

Our pets give us unconditional love and loyalty and we should pay just as much attention to their diet and care as we do our own. Animals respond to the use of herbs better than humans do. Almost any herbal treatment that is fit for human use can be used for your pets. Reduce the dosage to adjust for the difference in size (your pets are usually smaller than you are) and give the herbs in capsule form. Capsules may take a little longer to work, but keep the treatment going until your pet shows improvement.

PET TONIC: Thoroughly mix together the following: 1 pint of vinegar, 4 tablespoons cod-liver oil, 2 tablespoons of garlic powder, 5 tablespoons desiccated liver powder, and 4 tablespoons bone meal powder. Store in the refrigerator and give 3 tablespoons daily, in their food. Dogs love this.

TONIC FOR PETS: Mix together 2 tablespoons each of burdock root, garlic powder, and cayenne pepper, and add 4 tablespoons of goldenseal powder. Fill some #0 capsules with the herbal mixture. Give your pet 1 capsule for each 10 pounds of weight every 4 hours. Continue treatment until capsules are gone.

FENUGREEK TONIC: Nothing is better to give your pet or farm animal then fenugreek tea. Place 2 teaspoons of fenugreek seeds in 1 cup of boiling water. Allow to steep 15 minutes. Strain and add at least once a week to their drinking water. Removes excess mucus from all the systems.

TONIC FOR BIRDS: Canaries and parakeets love to eat shepherd's purse. Simply break off the top flowering stem and place in the cage. Very good tonic.

CANARY AID: Add a dash of saffron to your canary's drinking water. This is said to help them sing more. Saffron is a stimulant so it sure would make them feel more like singing.

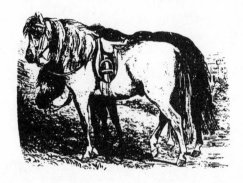

TONIC FOR HORSES: Allow the animal to eat several quarts of hops. Very good as a general tonic. Also calms a nervous animal.

VITAMIN FOOD FOR YOUR PET: Cook leftover turkey or chicken bones, or just cook a pound of liver. Add chopped onion, chopped celery, carrots or almost any vegetable. I've even added leftover spinach. Cook until the liver is done or the meat falls off the bones. Remove the bones from the liquid and reheat the broth.

Stirring constantly, add white cornmeal to the mixture by the handful until the mixture is very thick. You will hardly be able to stir it. Pour into large pans that have been rinsed with cold water. You can add garlic powder to the mixture if you like. Slice when cool. The animals love it. We fry up the liver mush and serve with maple syrup for our breakfast.

BIRD CAKES: We feel it is important to feed our wild friends. Mix together 1 cup of peanut butter, 2 cups wild bird seed, 5 cups corn meal, and 1 cup melted suet. Spoon into paper lined muffin tins. Add a string to the middle of each "muffin" if you plan to hang them up in trees. Refrigerate until used.

LINIMENT FOR LEG STRAINS: Bring 1 quart of cider vinegar to a gentle boil. Add 2 tablespoons of cayenne pepper and continue to gently boil for 10 minutes. Apply to the area needed twice daily. This increases stimulation to the area. It is good to use when treating horses for leg strains (if they're not too serious). It can also be applied to the chest area for congestion and colds.

RHEUMATISM TREATMENT FOR YOUR PET: Put 6 drops of oil of rosemary in 1/2 cup of water. Use this to massage the area that needs pain relief.

RHEUMATISM IN OLDER DOGS: Take a pillow that your dog sleeps on and stuff it with dried male fern leaves. This not only alleviates pain for the dog, it will also discourage fleas.

BED FLEAS: Sprinkle the bed with lavender oil and place fresh fennel under the bedding. Bugs hate the smell of fennel, so plant plenty near your kennel area. You can also stuff your pet's pillow with pennyroyal, eucalyptus, peppermint, red cedar shavings, rue, or sassafras shavings.

FLEA POWDER: Mix and grind 1 cup each of rue, wormwood, rosemary, fennel, and peppermint. When the herbs have been ground to a powder, dust the animal with the herbal mixture, working it in as you go.

FLEA POWDER: Mix together 1 ounce each of powdered wormwood and rosemary. Add 2 ounces of powdered pennyroyal, and 2 teaspoons of cayenne pepper. Use as often as you would a commercial flea powder. Be careful—DO NOT GET THIS IN THE ANIMAL'S EYES.

SURE FIRE WAY TO STOP FLEAS: Give your dog 1 tablet of 100 mg thiamine daily. I keep several outdoor cats and I grind 1 tablet daily and add this to their food. It works.

CAT PILLOW FLEA REPELLENT: Mix equal parts of chamomile and catnip. Add twice as much pennyroyal. Stuff a pillow with these herbs and they will love you.

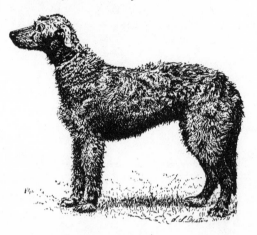

FLEA WASH: Add 1 cup fresh or dried rosemary to 1 quart of boiling water. Cover and steep until cool. Strain. Wash the dog and rinse well. Pour the herbal liquid on the dog and work in well. Leave the rosemary tea on the dog and let it dry.

DRY SHAMPOO FOR YOUR PETS: Split a vanilla bean and place it in 1 quart of orris root powder or cornmeal. Cover and let sit for 1 week. Sprinkle over the animal and brush it in thoroughly. Then brush it out.

TICKS: To remove ticks from you or your pet, dip a cotton swab in alcohol. Touch the tick and it should be easy to remove. Never touch the tick with your fingers, always use a pair of tweezers to remove it.

HOT SPOTS ON SPAYED FEMALE DOGS: Rub the affected area with wormwood oil. Repeat as necessary. Give them plenty of brewer's yeast with their meals.

HOT SPOTS: Mix equal parts olive oil and oil of thyme. Apply to the area with a cotton ball. This will stop the itching and prevent infections from starting in the areas they scratched before.

HAIR LOSS IN DOGS: Sprinkle goldenseal on the animals' feed and in their water. Do not use too much goldenseal. You can also make a weak solution of goldenseal tea and apply it to the area affected by hair loss. The animal will probably lick the solution off, but that's fine. Just make the solution weak, whether for internal or external use.

FLEA REPELLENT: This is also good for treating mange. I have never used this, but those that have swear by it. Simply apply WD-40 to the spine of the animal. It runs down the sides of the animal and keeps fleas away.

MANGE TREATMENT: Mange is caused by mites. Humans can contract mange from their pets, but is known as scabies in humans. It is a communicable disease, so be sure to treat your pet at the first sign of mange. The symptoms are the loss of hair and itching. Check your other pets if you find one that does have the disease. Mix 2 tablespoons each of garlic powder and goldenseal powder. Add to 1/4 cup of olive oil. Apply frequently to affected area.

MANGE TREATMENT: Another treatment for mange is used motor oil. It can be messy, but I have had people tell me that it works. Just pour the oil on the parts affected. Keep the pet as clean as possible and you should have no problem with mange. If the animal stays out of doors, make sure that the area where they sleep is kept clean.

EYE WASH: Put 2 tablespoons of comfrey root and 2 tablespoons bruised fennel seeds in 1 cup of water. Bring to a boil and remove from heat. Steep until cool. Keep refrigerated and use by putting in the eye with an eye dropper.

ANIMAL EAR CARE: Clean the ears of your pets by dipping a cotton swap in wormwood oil. This should prevent any problems with ear mites.

ANIMAL CUTS AND SCRAPES: Put a large handful of spearmint or peppermint in a container and cover with white vinegar. Allow to steep for 2 weeks. Strain. Apply to any sores on the animal or use to clean an area after the animal has had surgery. Stops the wound from itching while healing and the animal is less apt to scratch the area and tear the wound open again.

SORE FOOT PADS: Split an aloe vera leaf and rub on the pads of the dog's foot. Massage in thoroughly and reapply frequently.

CAT TOY: Cats love the smell of valerian. Stuff a toy mouse and they will become quite frisky. Horses also enjoy the smell, and will try to reach for it. Valerian has a calming effect on most animals and they will become playful when given a chance to calm down. Many people use it to bait mouse traps, as mice too enjoy the plant.

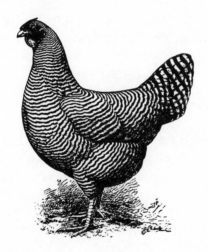

TO KEEP CHICKENS LICE FREE: Place wood ashes in a pile in the chicken yard. The chickens love to use this as a dust bath and it keeps them free of lice.

WORM TREATMENT: Getting your pet to take garlic every day may be a problem. Try this remedy every month or so for an easier way to keep your pet worm-free. Put 4 cloves of chopped garlic in a pan and pour 1 cup of boiling water over the garlic and let it sit overnight. After straining the liquid, mix with your dog's dry food the next day and give smaller amounts of food then normal to ensure that the animal eats all the food.

WORMWOOD TREATMENT FOR INTERNAL PARASITES: Have the animal go without food for 24 hours before treatment. Mix together 1 tablespoon each of powdered garlic, wormwood and thyme. After mixing well, fill #0 capsules with herbal mixture. Give the animal 1 capsule for every 10 pounds of weight. Give the dose every four hours during the day. Give the dog a mild dose of castor oil twice a day—in the morning and in the evening, the same day of treatment. If your dog has worms, I suggest that you bury the feces so that your pet does not get reinfested. To help soothe and calm the animal, give your dog some water with a bit of catnip tea in it.

WORMING YOUR HORSE OR GOAT: They really start begging for this. Give each animal several non-filter cigarettes each week. Keeps them from getting worms.

WORMING SWINE: Leave small lumps of coal in the pen. They will eat what they need to keep worm free.

KEEP SWINE FROM BITING EACH OTHER: Pigs are intelligent animals and get bored easily unless they are kept busy. They may have a tendency to bite the tails off of each other. Put toys in the pen for them to play with. Give them things that they can push around and get rough with. Old tires are good playthings for them. Look around and I'm sure you can find different things that you can put in with them.

My goats used to enjoy playing with a beach ball. They really kept busy with it. A beach ball would not last long with pigs, but there are other things you can use. I've even put in a sturdy wagon and they push that around.

SCOURS IN GOATS: Feed them as much fresh purslane as they will eat. This can also be made into a tea and used to stop diarrhea in humans.

WINDY COLIC IN ANIMALS: Give the animal plenty of angelica to eat. This should give relief within hours.

WINDY COLIC TREATMENT: Pour 1 quart of boiling water over 4 tablespoons of bruised caraway seeds and simmer for 30 minutes. Strain and add to the animals drinking water. Should give relief within 15 minutes. Fennel seed can also be used, as it too is good for treating windy colic.

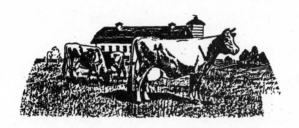

TO STIMULATE MILK PRODUCTION: This is a good tea to give cows and goats in order to stimulate milk production. Put a large handful of holy thistle in a bucket of water. Let sit overnight. Strain and give the animal the tea to drink in the morning. This keeps the animal calm and this helps to increase milk.

SORE TEATS: Melt 1/2 ounce of beeswax in a cup of almond oil. Apply daily. If the teats are cracked, add 1 cup of calendula to 1 cup of almond oil and allow to steep 24 hours. Strain and then add 1/2 ounce of melted beeswax to the oil mixture. Stir continuously while cooling. Apply several times daily.

TO TREAT MASTITIS: Mix slippery elm powder with enough water to form a paste. Apply to a clean cloth and apply to the affected area.

MASTITIS TREATMENT: Mastitis is an inflammation of the teat. Entry of the germ may be through the nipple. There are often cracks and abrasions of the nipple. It can also be caused by retention of milk. The disease may cause distention of the bag and can be very painful.

Washing the nipples before milking and being very clean in caring for your animals helps to prevent diseases. Adding a good softening cream to the nipples helps to keep them healthy. Clean the area thoroughly with a strong thyme tea. Apply a hot compress of thyme tea to the teat. Add 1/4 cup of dried thyme to 2 cups boiling water. Steep 30 minutes. Strain and reheat. Dip the cloth in the herbal liquid and apply as a compress. Repeat as necessary.

PROTECT GRAIN FOR LIVESTOCK: To keep bugs from the grain, add a cheesecloth bag full of bay leaves to the grain barrel.

FLY REPELLENT: Pennyroyal makes an effective and safe fly repellent for livestock. Put a large handful of pennyroyal in a pint of water. Boil for 5 minutes. Mix the herbal liquid with equal amounts of mineral oil. Add a few drops of dishwashing liquid and shake vigorously. Spray on the animal, in the stalls and on the wood around the barn door.

BASIL FLY REPELLENT: To help keep flies from the barn, plant plenty of sweet basil around the barn area. Planting it close to the house will help keep flies away from there, too.

TO GET RID OF MICE IN THE BARN OR HOUSE: Fill 1 bowl with water and another bowl with dried instant mashed potatoes. They eat the dry potatoes and then drink the water. This causes them to bloat and they will die.

MICE REPELLENT: Add 1 tablespoon of Tabasco sauce and 1/2 cup of soap detergent to 1 gallon of water. Use this to spray around the bottom of the barn—inside and out—to repel mice.

CAT AND DOG REPELLENT: There are areas that your pet is not welcome to invade. Cats can't stand the smell of ginger, so sprinkle that around your flower beds. Cayenne pepper is another good spice to use in keeping your pets from garden and flower beds. Once they get a whiff of the cayenne pepper they do not return.

GARDEN TIPS

DEER REPELLENT: Mix 1/2 tablespoon of dried blood to each gallon of water. Use this as a spray to keep deer away from plants and shrubs. This will also work to keep rabbits from the garden area. Just spray around the edge of the garden. You can find dried blood at your garden store. It is a fertilizer made from evaporated blood and nonfatty refuse from slaughterhouses.

RABBIT REPELLENT: Add cow manure to water and pour it over plants that you want protected. It also works to pour the manure tea around the edge of the garden, although I like to give the plants a fertilizer boost with the manure tea while protecting them from rabbits.

MOLE CONTROL: Plant castor beans around the edge of your garden to keep moles away.

MOLES: If moles are a problem in your garden, try planting Mexican marigold as a cover crop. Turn it under in the fall for a really great soil cleanser and a good green manure. They also repel rabbits, along with any soil borne pests.

CONTROL JAPANESE BEETLES: Garlic planted around the edge of your garden will discourage Japanese beetles. Castor beans will also work to help discourage them, as well as keeping moles away.

CONTROLS MOTHS AND WORMS: Pouring soured milk on cabbage and other plants will discourage moths and cabbage worms.

HOOKWORM: Plant dill and\or borage with your tomatoes to repel hookworms.

ROSE CARE: Turnips and anise, planted around the roses, will discourage aphids and spider mites.

ROSE CARE: Put tobacco in the blender and add water. Blend well and use this as a spray to control aphids.

ROSE CARE: Put several cloves of garlic in the blender with water. Blend well and use as a spray to control aphids.

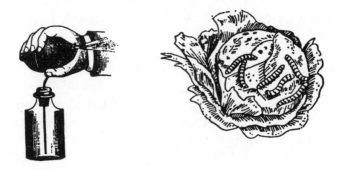

MAKE YOUR OWN DORMANT INSECT OIL SPRAY: Mix together 1 cup of liquid detergent, 1/2 cup of fish oil and 1/2 cup of number 10 mineral oil. Add the oil mixture to 2 gallons of water in a steady small stream, stirring constantly. Pour into sprayer and you're ready to go to work. It's good to control aphids, eggs of coddling moths, fruit moths, cankerworms, scale and a lot of other sucking and chewing insects that bother your fruit trees.

TO INHIBIT FUNGAL SPORES THAT AFFECT GERMINA-TION: Put equal parts of clematis, corn leaves, and the outer papery shell of garlic in the blender. Add enough water to cover and blend at high speed. Strain and spray affected plants until the fungus goes away.

·13·

Household and Family Tips

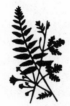

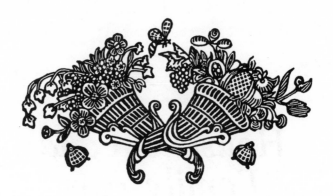

The house is the center of good family relations. Being creative with certain problems in a natural way helps us to appreciate the home even more. Part of that appreciation means finding ways to keep busy and happy. I have added projects to keep children busy learning new things during those rainy days, or just days when parents are busy with other chores. Some of these games and projects will be as fun for adults as they are for children, so some of those chores just might get put off for another day. Fun time spent with your children is time well spent.

I really feel that being a mother is the most important job in the world. A good start during infancy and the early years of childhood sets the stage for adulthood, so I have included a few special recipes for nursing mothers. I feel that breast-feeding is the only way to go, so the recipes deal with increasing milk production. I breast-fed my first two children, but unfortunately the last two were born a few months prematurely, so the opportunity was not there.

Part of having a well-run home is being prepared for emergencies—and I consider unexpected guests an emergency. Many of our friends drop by unexpectedly, but no one ever leaves my home without eating a good meal. My parents were sticklers about that and I guess I keep the same hospitality rules in my house.

In addition to eating a good meal, my guests leave with new knowledge about some delicious and nutritious wild plants. Many of them tell me they enjoy eating with us because they never know what I'm serving next. I take that as a compliment. Keep them surprised and you keep them interested.

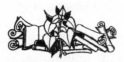

There are many jobs around the house that we all have to do. Here are a few hints on how to do them in a more natural way.

KEEP FRESH CUT FLOWERS LONGER: Add 2 tablespoons of lemon juice and 1 tablespoon of sugar to 1 quart of water. Add 1/2 teaspoon of bleach and your flowers will stay fresh much longer.

OVEN CLEANER: Sprinkle water on the bottom of the oven. Put baking soda in an even layer over the water. Sprinkle again with water and let sit overnight. Wipe off with a clean, damp cloth.

MILDEW TREATMENT: Wash down the areas that are prone to mildew with a strong thyme tea. Steep 1 quart of thyme in 1 gallon of water for several days. Use to scrub down the area.

TOILET BOWL CLEANER: Drop 3 vitamin C capsules in the bowl and let sit overnight. Scrub with brush in the morning. Stains are gone.

TOILET BOWL CLEANER: Drop several tablets of denture cleaner in the bowl and let sit overnight. Scrub with brush and stains are gone.

ROOM FRESHENER: To freshen the air while you vacuum, simply soak a cotton ball with your favorite scented oil and add to your vacuum cleaner bag. The whole house will smell wonderful.

AIR FRESHENER: This will clean your aluminum pots while freshening the air in your house at the same time. Drop slices of grapefruits, lemons or oranges in your pot. Cover with water and simmer for an hour.

ROOM FRESHENER: Add 3 pounds of green spruce tree cones to 4 gallons of water. Let steep for at least 24 hours. Boil the mix for 2 hours. Add to humidifier. This can also be added to the bath water for treatment of rheumatic discomforts.

ROMANTIC ROOM FRESHENER: Place several drops of your favorite scented oil on the light bulbs. The heat from the bulbs will make the fragrance fill the air.

CLOSET FRESHENER: Saturate a cotton ball in your favorite scented oil and place on a shelf in the closet. Repeat as needed.

KITCHEN REFRESHER: I use dishwashing liquid to mop my kitchen floor because it adds a shine to the floor and is easy to rinse. Add scented oil to your mop water for a fragrant kitchen. I add peppermint oil around Christmas. Any of the scents really add a lot to your home. The floral scents are good to use in the spring and summer. The cooking spices, such as cinnamon or nutmeg, are good for fall and winter.

I really like the fragrance of vanilla and add vanilla incense oil to my cleaning water. After using a certain fragrance for all your cleaning needs over a period of time, the whole house holds a permanent fragrance.

DRAIN MAINTENANCE: Pour 1/2 cup of baking soda down the drain. Pour in 1/2 cup of lemon juice or vinegar. Wait 15 minutes before flushing with hot water.

WALL PAPER CLEANER: Use slices of white bread to clean wall paper. Just wipe away the stains and dirt with the bread.

FLOOR WAX: Melt 4 tablespoons of paraffin and add to 2 quarts of mineral oil. Cool before storing in glass bottle. Apply to floor and allow to dry 30 minutes before lightly buffing.

WOODEN FLOOR POLISH: Mix together 4 tablespoons gum arabic, 4 tablespoons turpentine, 1 quart denatured alcohol, and 1 cup of orange shellac. Stir until the gum arabic dissolves. Apply with a cloth and allow to dry for 30 minutes before buffing. This can be stored for later use, but be sure to label it. It gives a high shine and makes floors non-slip.

FURNITURE POLISH: Add 1 tablespoon of lemon oil to 1 quart of mineral oil. Place in a spray bottle and use on wooden furniture. Rub it in and then wipe off.

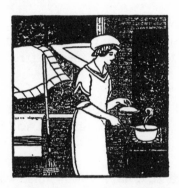

FURNITURE POLISH: Mix together 1 teaspoon of olive oil and 1/2 cup of lemon juice in a small pan. Dip a cloth in the liquid and wring out. Use this to dust and polish furniture. The cloth can be used repeatedly.

CHROME CLEANER: Cut a lemon in half. Wipe the chrome with the lemon.

METAL AND BRASS CLEANER: Horsetail is an excellent herb for cleaning metal because of it's high content of silica. Simply rub the metal with the fresh herb. Or, make a strong tea and soak the metal in it. To make the tea, add 1 quart of horsetail (packed) to 1 quart of water and boil it. Allow it to sit overnight. Immerse the metal in the tea.

LAUNDRY BLEACH: Add 1/4 cup of vinegar to your wash. Removes odor along with dirt.

REMOVE GREASE FROM CLOTHING: Cola soft drink may be corrosive to your body's system, but it does get the grease out of your clothes. Pour 1 can of cola in your washer when you need to clean really greasy clothes. Dissolves the grease fast. (Edgar Cayce recommended drinking 1 can a month to clean your system.)

FABRIC SOFTENER: Using fabric softener on bed linen and clothing of asthmatic people can sometimes cause asthma attacks. It's best to line dry all clothing and linens. Do not use fabric softener.

MAKE YOUR OWN LYE: Place wood ashes in a pan of water and allow to soak overnight. Strain off the wood ashes and you have the lye water. Use it to make soap. (See soap recipes in chapter four "Skin Problems.")

BUG FREE GRAIN AND FLOUR: Add bay leaves to a small bag of pepper (black or cayenne) and tie tight. Add to flour bin to keep out the weevils.

SILVERFISH: Place costmary sprigs (also called "Bible leaf") around the house to get rid of silverfish.

FLY REPELLENT FOR PICNICS: Leave freshly picked basil on the picnic table to keep your picnic free of flies. For protection inside of the house, put basil sprays all around in the rooms. Chamomile, garlic, and mints are good to leave lying around the house as they are all good bug chasers. Yarrow repels many insects if used as a spray.

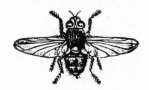

FLY REPELLENT: Crunch equal amounts of bay leaves, crushed cloves, pennyroyal, and eucalyptus. Place in attractive mesh bags and hang close to doors or on your screen door.

ANT REPELLENT: Place goldenseal tea bags around the area where there are ants. They soon leave.

ANT REPELLENT: Place crushed catnip on ant trails. They will leave the house.

KEEPS INSECTS FROM THE HOUSE: Hang dried bunches of tomato leaves in each room of the house. Keeps insects away.

MOTH REPELLENT: Hang bunches of sage in your closet to keep moths away.

WORM TREATMENT FOR CHILDREN: Have the child eat 1/2 cup of blackberries with each meal for 3-4 days. This will dispel the worms.

HEAD LICE: Pour 1 quart of boiling water over 1 large handful of tobacco leaves. Let steep several hours. Strain, keeping the liquid. You will need to reuse this tobacco rinse, so have a basin ready to catch the liquid as you pour it directly over freshly shampooed hair. Rinse the hair in it at least 15 times. Comb hair directly after rinsing. Leave on for several hours before shampooing out.

I have had people tell me that they used the tobacco from a pack of cigarettes (they removed the papers) and this worked very well.

INSECT REPELLENT: Rub oil of sassafras on the skin before venturing out. To make it, put 1 cup of sassafras into a jar and cover it with vodka. Screw the lid on tightly. Put it out in the sun for the whole day, or in a low heat oven overnight. I set mine on top of our baseboard heater.

INSECT REPELLENT: Put 2 tablespoons oil of pennyroyal in 2 cups of vodka. Shake well and apply to skin before going outdoors.

STOP HICCUPS: Eat 1 teaspoon of sugar. Should stop hiccups immediately.

EXPOSURE TO NUCLEAR ACCIDENT: Chew 4 dolomite tablets 4 times daily. The pectin found in apples is also good to use. Pulverize 3 apples and eat 3 apples at least 4 times daily. Both these methods help to bind strontium and carry it from the system.

APPETITE SUPPRESSANT: Rub a clove of garlic on your upper lip before eating.

CATTAILS: Cattails are good for making gifts or for home use. Break them up and they make wonderful stuffing for quilts. They are insulating, so they really keep you warm. You can also use them to line coats or vests. They are good to use in hunting coats as they are waterproof and insulate for warmth while out in the cold.

HINTS FOR NURSING MOTHERS
FENNEL TEA FOR NURSING MOTHERS: Fennel tea is good for milk production. Pour 1 cup boiling water over 1 teaspoon of dried fennel. Steep 5 minutes. Strain and sweeten. You can add a dash of ginger if desired.

BORAGE TEA FOR NURSING MOTHERS: Use borage flowers and leaves to make this tea. Put 1/4 cup of chopped leaves and flowers in 2 cups boiling water. Allow to steep 10 minutes. Strain and sweeten. Drink several cups a day. This is also good to soothe nerves, while helping to increase milk production.

SWEET BASIL TO INCREASE MILK PRODUCTION: Add 2 teaspoons of sweet basil to 1 cup of boiling water. Steep 10 minutes and strain. Sweeten and drink several times daily.

INCREASE MILK PRODUCTION: Add 2 tablespoons of hops and 1 teaspoon of violet flowers to 1 cup boiling water. Steep 10 minutes. Strain and sweeten with honey. Drink several times a day. Also helps to relax Mother.

DRY UP MOTHER'S MILK: Put 2 teaspoons of sage in 1 cup of milk and simmer gently for 10 minutes. Strain and sweeten with honey. Drink several times daily.

PREGNANCY: Red raspberry tea is said to make birthing easier if used throughout the pregnancy. Pick 4-5 fresh leaves and pour 1 cup boiling water over the leaves. Cover and steep for 10 minutes. Strain and sweeten.

THINGS TO KEEP THE KIDS BUSY

GROWING COALS: This is something fun for the kids to do. Place several chunks of coal in a deep dish. Mix together 2 tablespoons of water, 1 tablespoon of bluing, 1 tablespoon ammonia, and 2 tablespoons of salt. Pour over the coal. Put several drops of different colors of food coloring at different places on the coal. It will take several days before the coal starts growing.

ELDER FLUTE: To entertain children while you are berry picking, hollow out a small branch of the elder to create a musical instrument. They become quite creative with it.

FINGER PAINTS: Mix 2 cups cold water with 1/4 cup of cornstarch. Add food coloring. You can also store this in the refrigerator for later use.

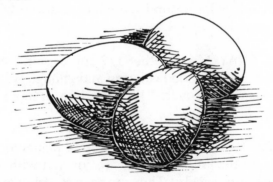

EASTER EGGS: This is the old fashioned way to color eggs. Wrap the eggs with onion skins and wrap in foil. The eggs come out golden. Use beeswax to put names or designs on the eggs. While you are writing on the eggs, place brown or red onion skins in an old pan and cover with water. Heat the water to boiling. Add designed eggs and boil slowly for 30 minutes. Remove and dry.

An easier and more interesting way is to raise Araucana chickens. They lay colored eggs. If you breed an Araucana rooster with a Rhode Island Red hen, the offspring will lay pink eggs. You will have varying shades of pink, blue and green eggs. Kids don't fuss much about caring for these chickens. They are very mild tempered and the eggs are said to be lower in cholesterol.

BASKET DYE: Kids love to make gifts. Teach them to make small baskets and to use natural dyes to color them. Walnut is one of the easiest natural dyes to make. Put walnut hulls in water and simmer for several hours. Dip the baskets in the liquid and the basket becomes very pleasing to look at. This makes a useful gift, one that can be kept forever.

If you want your baskets to be scented, soak the reeds in an essential oil for 15 minutes. This will also keep the reed supple while you're working with it. The basket will give off a pleasant scent.

GIFT IDEA: To make attractive book marks, dry an herb of your choice between absorbent paper. Press it flat with something heavy. When dry, place between two pieces of plastic. You can cut the plastic into a shape or design that you find pleasing. Anchor with glue, punch holes around the edge, and lace with yarn or embroidery thread.

MODELING CLAY: Mix together 1/2 cup of salt, 1 cup flour, 3 teaspoons of alum. Add food coloring and enough water to make a nice clay. Keep in a covered jar, kneading in more water if it becomes too dry.

JOB'S TEARS: Job's Tears make interesting plants for your children to grow. In the fall, the plants are covered with hard beads that make beautiful jewelry. They are easy to string and children enjoy making their own gifts. To string the beads, use fishing line. It makes a strong necklace.

FOOD RECIPES

I've included a few recipes that are easy to make and can be used in emergencies. Sometimes, unexpected company stops over and you have to be ready to fix meals quickly. Some of these recipes are just plain handy to have around; they help with your food budget.

Make sure that the wild plants and herbs mentioned in some of the recipes are ones that you are familiar with before attempting to use them. Herb identification books are helpful. You can have a lot of fun purchasing books by experts, books that could lead you to a whole new interest in gathering wild foods. You could check with your public library for some of the books. I like to buy the books so that I have them around for reference. I take a field guide with me whenever I go out to forage for wild plants or mushrooms.

There are gardening groups that give walks and talks on wild foods. You will meet many knowledgeable people through such a group. Becoming interested in wild foods can lead you in a whole new direction. I also think that knowing about any subject is great, just for the sake of learning. That knowledge could be of help to you in the future.

MAKE YOUR OWN COFFEE SUBSTITUTE: Use either dandelion or chicory root. Wash the roots carefully and spread in a large flat pan. Place in an oven at 180 to 200 degrees for up to 4 hours. Turn to ensure even drying. When the roots are completely dry and cool, you may store them as roots to grind fresh, or you could grind them before placing in a tightly closed container. Use as you would coffee, or mix half and half with commercial coffee.

CORN COFFEE: Put dried corn in a pan. Add boiling water and continue boiling for 5 minutes. Sweeten with maple syrup. This was a favorite of the Iroquois Indians.

ANOTHER COFFEE SUBSTITUTE: Mix and grind together 1 cup of ginseng root, 1/2 cup licorice root, 1 cup sarsaparillas root, 1 cup Irish moss, 2 cups of holy thistle, 1/2 cup dried orange peel, and 5 cups roasted chicory or dandelion root. Use powdered malt in place of licorice root if you desire.

SWISS MOCHA: Mix together 1/2 cup of instant coffee, 2 tablespoons cocoa, 1/3 teaspoon baking soda, 1 cup sugar, and 1 cup dried milk. Blend in the blender until very fine. Place 2 teaspoons of mixture in 1 cup boiling water.

INTERNATIONAL COFFEE: Mix together 1 cup instant coffee, 2 cups powdered coffee creamer, 1 teaspoon of cinnamon, 1 cup of sugar, and 2 cups of powdered milk. Place in blender and mix until very fine. Use 2 or more teaspoons to each cup of boiling water.

CAFE VIENNA: Mix together in blender: 1/2 cup instant coffee, 1/2 teaspoon cinnamon, pinch of baking soda, 2/3 cup of powdered milk, and 2/3 cup of sugar. Blend until fine. Use 2 rounded teaspoons for each cup of boiling water.

CAFE CAPPUCCINO: Mix in the blender until fine, 1 cup powdered milk, 3/4 cup sugar, 1/2 cup instant coffee, 1/4 teaspoon dried or powdered orange peel and 1/8 teaspoon of baking soda. Add 2 rounded teaspoons to each cup of boiling water.

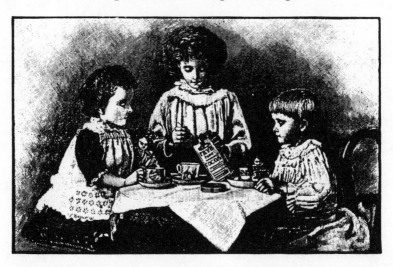

HOT CHOCOLATE: Mix together in blender until fine, 2 cups of powdered milk, 1 cup powdered sugar, 1/4 cup of cocoa, 1 cup of powdered coffee creamer, and a dash of salt. If you like, you can add 2 tablespoons of malted milk power. To use, add 4 tablespoons of mixture to 1 cup of boiling water.

MINTED HOT CHOCOLATE: Prepare your hot chocolate. Stir it with a peppermint candy stick.

MAKE YOUR OWN SWEETENED CONDENSED MILK: Mix together 2/3 cup of sugar, 1 cup powdered coffee creamer, 1/2 cup of boiling water and 3 tablespoons of margarine. Blend in blender until smooth. Use in any recipe that calls for sweetened condensed milk.

HOT MULLED PUNCH: This is good to make for large gatherings. Add 1-1/2 quarts of cranberry juice to 2 quarts of apple juice. Put in a 36 to 40 cup coffee maker. Place 1/2 cup of brown sugar, 1-1/2 teaspoons of whole cloves and about 4-5 cinnamon sticks in the basket of the coffee maker. When cycle is done, remove the basket containing the spices and serve hot. Very festive and good.

BORAGE JUICE HELPER: Wash several leaves of borage and place in blender. Add enough water to cover and blend at high speed until mixture is smooth. Add to iced tea or any drink for added vitamins. Kids love the taste.

APPLE TEA: This is good to keep handy as you will use it to treat many illnesses, although you can drink it just for enjoyment. Wash and core several apples and slice, do not peel. Put the apples on a greased, waxpaper-lined cookie sheet. Place in an oven on low heat, with door cracked open. Turn over to ensure they dry completely. When apple slices are dry, close oven door and roast until lightly browned. Cool and store in tightly closed container. Place several slices in your teapot and fill with boiling water. Steep about 10 minutes. Add honey as needed for sweetener. This is a real good tonic for the kidneys.

FRESH LEMON BALM TEA: Take 20 sprigs of fresh lemon balm, 4 tablespoons honey, 10 whole cloves, and the juice of 1/2 lemon. Pour 1 quart of boiling water over the lemon balm, then add the other ingredients. Let steep 10 minutes. Strain and serve.

ROSE HIP TEA: Gather and clean the rose hips. Chop in the blender. Air dry them before storing in a tightly closed container. To make the tea, pour 1 cup boiling water over 1/2 teaspoon of the crushed rosehips. Steep 5 minutes until color is bright pink. Add sugar or honey. For added taste, try it with cloves, or use cinnamon sticks to stir the tea.

ROSE HIP WINE: After cleaning them thoroughly, crush 5 pounds of rosehips. Place in 2 quarts of water and allow to sit overnight. Add 1 ounce of yeast and 1-3/4 pounds of sugar. Let ferment for 7 days. Strain well. Add 2 quarts of water, and an additional 1-3/4 pounds of sugar. Allow to ferment again. This makes a good heart tonic and is delicious.

SURVIVAL FOOD: The young flower heads of sunflowers can be boiled in water and eaten like brussel sprouts. Grind the seeds from sunflowers and add to breads, soups, and cakes for extra vitamins.

MILKWEED: Milkweed is a very versatile plant. The shoots can be used as asparagus, the newly opened leaves as spinach. The unopened flower buds taste like broccoli.

The pods are cooked like okra. Just cover with boiling water and boil 1 minute. Drain and repeat 3 times, then boil for 10 minutes.

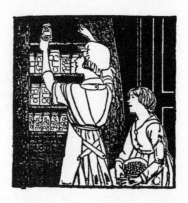

DRIED CORN: Cut 13 cups of corn from the cob. Add 1 cup of sugar and 1 cup of cream to the corn. Bring to a boil, stirring constantly. Place in shallow pans and allow to dry in a slow oven with the door cracked. Store in tightly closed container.

CARROT SUBSTITUTE: Use wild carrot roots (*Daucus carota*) in soups and stews. The soft tissue around the pith is the part to use. It is commonly known as Queen Anne's Lace. *Caution:* Be sure that it has the characteristic smell of carrot before using, as the plant does resemble hemlock, a deadly plant.

WILD ASPARAGUS: Pick when the spears first emerge. Steam the spears until tender. Put about 3 spears in a flour tortilla. Cover the spears with cheddar cheese and Miracle Whip. Place under broiler or in microwave until cheese is melted. Add fresh bean sprouts, roll up and enjoy.

CHICKWEED THICKENER: The seeds from chickweed can be used to thicken gravies and stews.

CHICKWEED PANCAKES: Blanch the leaves of chickweed for 3 minutes. Chop them up very fine in the blender and add to pancake mixture.

CHICKWEED SALAD HELPER: Chickweed flowers are an interesting ingredient to add to salads. You can use the young leaves in salads, too. Add the flowers and leaves to stews and soups.

CELERY SUBSTITUTE: The seeds from the head of wild celery (*Apium graveolens*) can be added to soups and stews to add a celery flavor.

GINGER CANDY: Boil the roots of wild ginger (*Asarum canadense*) until soft. Drain and add the roots to maple syrup and simmer. It's an unusual treat.

EASY SAUERKRAUT: Put a one-inch thick layer of shredded cabbage in an crock. Sprinkle with 1 teaspoon of salt. Continue to layer the cabbage and the salt until the crock is full. Place a plate over the sauerkraut and weigh down with something heavy. Let it sit overnight and remove the scum that will be on the top the next day. Stir the cabbage thoroughly. Do this daily until the fermentation has stopped. Place in sterile jars and cover tightly.

DANDELION WINE: When the dandelions are in full bloom and there is no rain or dew, pick 3 quarts of dandelion blossoms, packed tight. Wash them and place them in a crock. Pour 2 gallons of boiling water over the blossoms. Let stand 36 hours. Strain through a colander. Add 7 pounds of sugar.

Take 6 oranges and 6 lemons and roll them to make them juicier. Slice the lemons and oranges with the skins on. Add to the wine. Add 1/4 box of seedless raisins. Stir thoroughly. Let sit for another 24 hours. Add 1 cake of yeast or 1 envelope of dry yeast. Stir and strain through wet muslin or a clean dish towel. Pour into bottles with screw-on lids. Fill to brimming. Cover the bottles by tying pieces of muslin over the tops. Put aside in a cool place for 6 months. When fermentation is complete, (when no more bubbles appear in the bottles), you can screw on the lids.

CAROTENE ADDITION TO SALADS: Dock leaves have 4 times more carotene then carrots. When dock leaves are young and tender, add them to salads. Dry some to add to soups.

NATURAL THICKENER: Use arrowroot to thicken soups and gravies.

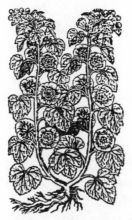

Hollyhock (Althea rosea)

HOLLYHOCK: Hollyhock is a member of the mallow family. The leaves can be eaten as a salad green or as a cooked green.

ROSE HIP SOUP: Cover 2 cups of rosehips with 2 cups of water and simmer 2 hours until rosehips are tender.

In a separate bowel, mix 1/2 cup of sugar with 2 tablespoons of cornstarch. Add this to the rose hip soup to thicken it. Boil briskly 3 minutes, stirring constantly. Add 1/2 cup of white wine before serving. If served cold, top with whipped cream and lemon slices.

MAKE YOUR OWN YOGURT: Dissolve 4 cups of dried milk in 3 cups of lukewarm water and add 1 can evaporated milk. In a separate bowel, dissolve 1 envelope gelatin in 1 cup of boiling water. Wait until the mixture is lukewarm, then mix the two together and add 4 tablespoons of plain yogurt. Make sure that the mixture is not over 100 degrees as it will kill the yogurt cultures if it gets any hotter.

Have the oven preheated to 250 degrees. Pour yogurt mixture into a glass container and place it in the preheated oven. Turn the oven off. Leave it in the oven for 24 hours. Remove from oven, place it in containers, and refrigerate.

You can add any fruit that you like to the yogurt. We love cherries. I add about 1/2 quart of canned cherries (I use the blender to get them finely chopped enough to stir into the yogurt.

Cherries are good for treating gout, so we make plenty to give my son-in-law, who suffers from gout. He eats it frequently. Plain yogurt is also used a lot around our home as I feel that it is important to our diet. It's good on baked potatoes, salads, and fruit salads.

FRENCH DRESSING: Combine in a quart jar and shake well: 1/4 cup of water, 1/2 cup of vinegar, 1-1/2 cups salad oil, 1 cup catsup, 2 teaspoons Worcestershire sauce, 1/2 cup of sugar, 1 teaspoon salt, 1 teaspoon pepper, a teaspoon of table mustard, and 1/2 teaspoon powdered garlic.

THOUSAND ISLAND DRESSING: Mix together 1/2 cup mayonnaise to 2 tablespoons catsup, 1 chopped hard-boiled egg, 1 tablespoon chopped sweet pepper, and 1 tablespoon relish. Mix well and chill thoroughly.

ANOTHER VERSION OF THOUSAND ISLAND DRESSING: Combine 1 cup mayonnaise, 1/4 cup of catsup, 1 chopped hard-boiled egg, 1 finely chopped onion, 1/3 cup of chopped olives, 1 teaspoon table mustard, 1/4 cup of chopped sweet pepper, 1/2 cup of finely chopped celery. Mix well and chill thoroughly.

RUSSIAN DRESSING: Mix together 3 rounded tablespoons of mayonnaise, 2 tablespoons catsup, 1 teaspoon horseradish, 1/4 teaspoon Worcestershire sauce, 1 tablespoon relish. Mix well and chill before serving.

TARTAR SAUCE: Mix together 3 heaping tablespoons mayonnaise, 1 finely chopped hard-boiled egg, and 1 tablespoon relish. Chill before serving.

CELERY SEED DRESSING: Mix in the blender together, 1 tablespoon of salt, 1 tablespoon of celery seed, 1 to 1-1/2 tablespoon dry mustard, 3/4 teaspoon paprika, 3/4 cup of vinegar, 1 cup of sugar, and 1/2 of a small onion. When blended well, add 2-1/4 cup vegetable oil in a steady stream to the mixture. Refrigerate.

CHILI SAUCE: Peel and chop 1 gallon tomatoes, add 1/2 cup of chopped onion, 1/2 cup chopped sweet peppers, 1/2 cup chopped red peppers, 5 teaspoons salt, 1/2 cup of brown sugar, 1/2 teaspoon cayenne pepper, 1 teaspoon nutmeg, 2 teaspoons ginger, 1 teaspoon cinnamon, 1 tablespoon mustard. Mix well and add 1 quart of vinegar and cook to desired consistency. Pour into sterile jars and seal.

MAYONNAISE: Combine 1 egg in blender with 3/4 teaspoon of salt, 1/4 teaspoon of paprika, 1/4 teaspoon dry mustard, 1 tablespoon vinegar, 1 tablespoon of lemon juice. Add 1/4 cup of vegetable oil and start blender. Then, add 3/4 cup of vegetable oil in a small steady stream to the mixture, until smooth.

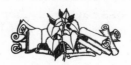

    I keep a few of these mixes around just because they are handy and great for emergency use. They can be stored and they keep forever. *Use dried herbs for these mixes.*

TACO MIX: Mix together 3 tablespoons each of oregano and corn starch, 2 tablespoons each of basil, crushed pepper flakes, and garlic powder. Add 5 tablespoons of chili pepper and 1/2 cup of minced onion flakes. Store in tightly closed container. Use 1-1/2 tablespoons of spice mix for each pound of meat. If making a meatless recipe, use 1-1/2 tablespoons of taco mix for every 2 cups of whatever you're using.

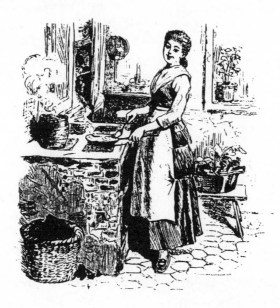

MAKE YOUR OWN POULTRY SEASONING: Mix together 3 tablespoons each of marjoram and thyme, and 1 tablespoon each of sage, savory and rosemary. Add 2 teaspoons of celery seeds, 1/2 teaspoon each of pepper, oregano, and allspice. Store in a tightly closed container and use in sauces, dressing, or any recipe where you would use poultry seasoning. This is good to add to meatloaf.

CURRY POWDER: Mix together 2 teaspoons coriander seeds, 4 teaspoons powdered cinnamon, 2 teaspoons ginger, 2 teaspoons ground turmeric. Mix together well and you have your own curry powder.

PICKLING SPICE: Mix together 2 tablespoons coriander seed, 2 tablespoons allspice, 1 tablespoon mustard seed, 2 bay leaves, and about 1 inch of a ginger root chopped fine.

PUMPKIN OR APPLE PIE SPICE: Mix together 3 teaspoons powdered allspice, 3 teaspoons nutmeg, 2 teaspoons ground cloves, 2 tablespoons cinnamon, and 2 tablespoons ground ginger. Store in jar with a tight lid.

CHICKEN SOUP SEASONING MIX: Mix together 1/4 cup each of chives, tarragon, marjoram, basil, savory and 3 teaspoons of sage. Add 1-2 teaspoons of the spice mix to your chicken soup. Store tightly closed. I put some of the dried mixes in a peppermill. This makes it easy to add the amount wanted for flavor.

PILAF RICE MIX: Mix together 3 tablespoons each of garlic powder and thyme, 2 teaspoons each of allspice and coriander, 1 tablespoon of black pepper, 5 tablespoons of oregano, and 3/4 cup of basil. Store in tightly closed container. Use 2 tablespoons of herb mixture for each cup of rice.

SCALLOPED POTATO MIX: Easy to store and easy to use. Mix together 16 tablespoons each of flour, cornstarch, and dried milk. Add 8 teaspoons of salt, 6 teaspoons onion powder and 1 teaspoon of pepper. Store in tightly closed container. To use, sprinkle 6 tablespoons of the mix over 3 cups of dehydrated potatoes. Dot with 3 tablespoons of butter, mix in 2-1/3 cups of boiling water and 2/3 cup of milk. Bake in a 350 degree oven for 50-55 minutes.

MAKE YOUR OWN DEHYDRATED POTATOES: Make this a family project and it goes pretty fast. Peel and slice potatoes. Blanch for 10 seconds. Place potatoes immediately in cold water and chill about 15 minutes. Dry off completely. Spray cookie sheet with vegetable oil cooking spray and place the sliced potatoes on the cookie sheets. Bake in oven set at 150 degrees. Prop open the oven door slightly. After about an hour, turn the slices over. It may take 3 hours to dry completely. They will be brittle when done. Cool and store in tightly closed container. Carrots can be dried in this manner also.

SOUP MIX: Mix together 8 teaspoons of instant bouillon (chicken or beef), 2 tablespoons of dried onion, and 1 teaspoon dried parsley. Store in tightly closed container. To use, add 2 tablespoons of the mix to 4 cups of water. Add other dried vegetables, such as dried diced carrots, mushroom slices, or other dried vegetables. Add as much rice or noodles as you desire. Simmer until rice or noodles are done. Add pepper as needed.

FRESH MUSTARD: To make your own flavors of mustard, start with mustard flour. To get English flavor, add vinegar. For Chinese flavor, use beer. You can also use white wine, horseradish, sage, oregano, paprika, basil, garlic, onion, chervil, cloves, lovage, turmeric, rosemary, marjoram, chili powder, cumin, allspice, cinnamon, thyme, tarragon, parsley, dill, Tabasco, curry, savory, nutmeg, or chives to flavor the mustard flour. Mix spices and the mustard flour in any combination before adding liquid. Thin with milk or mayonnaise. Add enough to make a smooth paste. Allow to stand until flavor is well blended. Mix in small batches for greater pungency. Keeps forever. Makes a nice gift.

MEATLESS PEAR MINCEMEAT: If you like the brand of None-Such prepared mincemeat, you will love this. It is the best recipe I've ever tasted for mincemeat. It calls for 10 large apples, 15 pounds of pears, 3 lemons, 3 boxes of seedless raisins (15 ounce boxes). Wash the pears; drain, peel, quarter, and core them. Wash the lemons and cut in quarters, removing seeds. Wash the apples; quarter and core, but do not peel. Alternately force pears, apples, lemons, raisins and 3 cups of walnuts through a food grinder, using a coarse blade. Combine fruit mixture with 5 pounds of sugar, 1-1/2 cups of white vinegar, 4 teaspoons each of ground cloves, cinnamon, nutmeg, and allspice in a large kettle. Bring to a boil over medium heat. Lower heat and simmer uncovered, stirring frequently for 40 minutes, or until mixture is thick. Pour at once into sterile jars, filling to 1/4 inch from top. Seal at once. Put the jars in a boiling water bath for 25 minutes. The recipe makes about 9 quarts.

MAPLE SYRUP: Stir together 4 cups of white sugar, 1/2 cup of brown sugar and 2 cups of water. Add 2 tablespoons of corn syrup if you have it. Cover and simmer for 10 minutes, Remove from heat and add 1 teaspoon of vanilla and 1 teaspoon maple flavoring. It's a quick syrup to make and it keeps well.

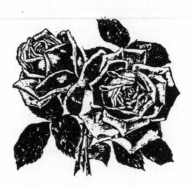

ROSE SYRUP: Boil 1 cup of water and 1 cup of sugar for 15 minutes. Add 1 cup fragrant red rose petals—petals only please. Steep until cool. Strain if desired. Use on pancakes, waffles or ice cream for a nice treat.

MAYAPPLE MARMALADE: Late summer or early fall, pick 1/2 gallon of ripe mayapples. *Remove the stem ends, as they are poisonous.* Cut in quarters and put in kettle. Add 1 cup of water and simmer for 15 minutes, stirring occasionally. When tender enough to mash, put through colander to remove the skins and seeds. To 4 cups of pulp add 1 box of pectin and bring to a boil. As soon as it comes to a boil add 5 cups of sugar. Stir constantly. Let it come to a hard boil and boil 1 minute. Remove from heat and skim off foam. Put into sterile jars immediately and seal. *Caution:* The plant is poisonous. Do not eat any of the leaves or stems from the plant. Collect the mayapples only when fully ripe. The American Indians used the young shoots to commit suicide, so you can see that it can be fatal.

DANDELION JELLY: Pick 1-1/2 quarts of dandelion blossoms. Take the stems off. Rinse the blossoms well. Add 3 cups of water and boil for about 3 minutes. Drain well and add 1 teaspoon of lemon extract, and 1/2 teaspoon of orange extract to 2-2/3 cup of the liquid. Mix in a box of pectin and bring to a rolling boil. Add 4-1/2 cups of sugar all at once to the mixture. Bring again to a boil and boil 3 minutes, stirring constantly. Remove from heat and skim off top. Put in sterile jars immediately and seal.

ROSE HIP MARMALADE: Pick and remove stem ends from 3 pounds of rosehips. Crush the hips in the blender. Place in pan and cover with 4 cups of boiling water and simmer 30 minutes. Rub through a sieve to remove seeds and hulls. This should yield about 5 cups of pulp.

Squeeze 2 large oranges and 1 lemon. Add the juices to the pulp. Put the rind of 1 orange through the grinder, add that to the pulp. Add 6 cups of sugar to the pulp mix. Boil about 20 minutes. Remove from heat, skim, and pour immediately in sterile jars, and seal.

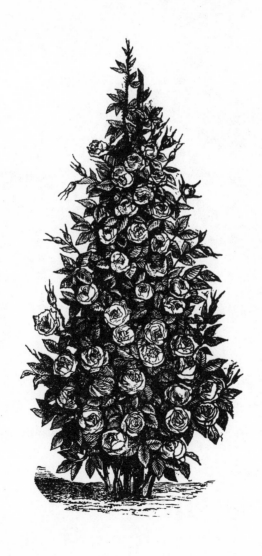

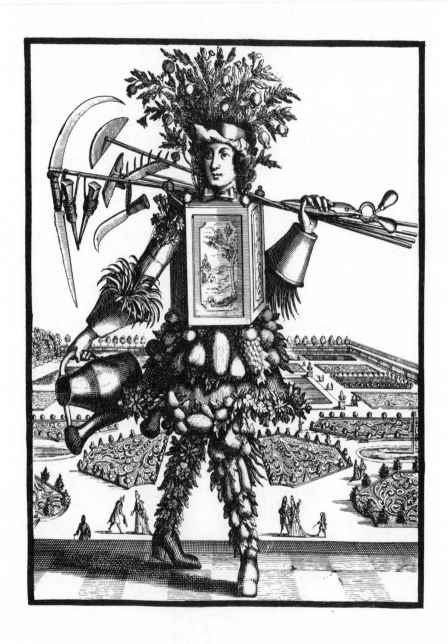

·14·

Harvesting the Herbs and Preparing Your Own Herbal Medicine Chest

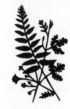

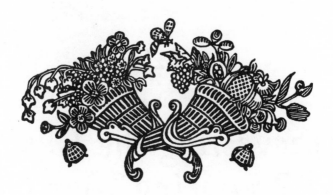

M ost of the time when you mention the word "herb," it means the part of the herb that grows above ground. Sometimes this means the entire plant growing above ground, but most of the time it means only the top half of the plant.

In general, herbs should be gathered when they are in flower. Never gather your herbs on a wet day. Always wait until there have been several dry days before collecting the herbs. Herbs should be gathered after the dew has dried from the plants, but before the sun gets too hot. They hold most of the essential aromatic oils at this time.

The leaves can be gathered when the plant is flowering. Hang up the stalks to air dry until the leaves are completely dry. You can then crumble the leaves, keeping only those leaves that retain a green color, and store in a dark, tightly closed container. The stems have very little medicinal value, so these need not be kept. Make sure the bunches of herbs hang loosely, so there is a chance for the air to circulate between the leaves. You do not want any mold to form on the leaves.

Some of the herbs need to be oven-dried to insure that they are dried as quickly as possible. This can keep the leaves from turning black. Basil is one of the herbs that needs to be dried quickly, to prevent it from turning black. Put a thin layer of the herb on a cookie sheet. Place in a very low-heat oven, about 150 degrees. Prop open the oven door with a spoon to release the moisture from the plants.

Turn the herbs and watch them carefully. Remove when the herb crumbles easily. Store in an airtight container immediately.

Some people are successful in drying their herbs in the microwave. I tried once and started a fire, because they do dry very quickly in the microwave. I never seem to have the time needed to stay close enough to make sure that they are drying correctly, so I use other methods. Maybe I can experiment with using the microwave next year. It would speed things up a bit, I'm sure.

The seeds of the herbs are gathered when they are not quite ripe, before the seed pods are fully opened. I pick the whole head of the plant and place it in a paper bag. I leave these to dry in the bag. When I happen to think of them, I shake the bag every once in a while. Later, I shake the bag to work the seeds loose from the pods. It is an easy matter to then pick out the flower heads, leaving the seeds at the bottom of the bag. I pour the seeds into a container and store them. It's easy.

The flowers of the herbs are collected just as they are beginning to open. These should be placed on a screen to dry. Lay them on the screen in a single layer and turn frequently until they are completely dry. They should retain a natural color, so keep only those that do keep their color.

When drying the fresh elder flowers, please take the precaution of hanging them away from people and living areas. They release a volatile gaseous oil that may cause you to become dizzy or give you a headache.

Most of the roots and bark are collected in the fall with a few exceptions. One exception is the wild ginger root. This should be gathered in the spring. As ginger is so necessary for cooking and medicinal purposes, I thought I would make a special mention of that. After getting a good patch of wild ginger to grow, you will be able to judge how much you can harvest without destroying your whole patch.

We need to preserve the wild plants around us. Never, never gather all of the wild herbs that you find. Always leave plenty for another year's supply. You need to be sure to leave plenty of plants alive to keep the species healthy and able to continue to grow where you found them. When gathering wild seed, it doesn't hurt

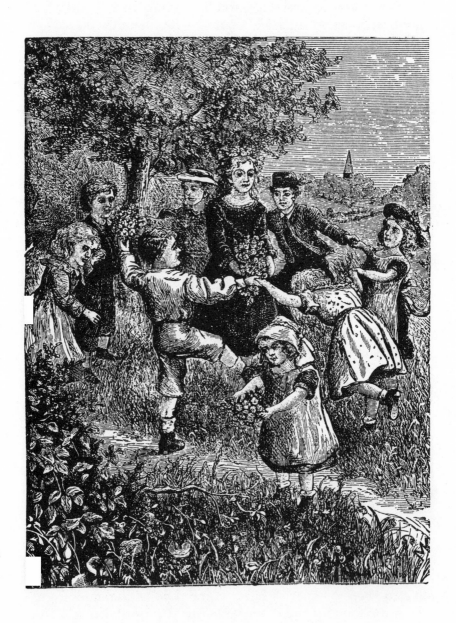

to plant a few seeds that you have gathered. I try to leave the stronger and healthier plants where I find them. The stronger plants insure that there will be a strong healthy patch a few years down the road.

I remember showing a friend the location of a patch of wild ginger. I never gathered from that patch, I was just attempting to teach her to identify the plant. The patch was growing in a protected area. The next time I saw the patch, it had been utterly destroyed. The "friend" thought she would dig up her supply so she dug enough to last for several years.

Since then, I have never attempted to teach anyone to identify the herbs again, except for the more common and easily found herbs, such as plantain, shepherd's purse, mullein and a few that are not in danger of being totally wiped out by someone who just does not have the proper mind set to appreciate these wild gifts.

If you can't find any sources from which to buy bark, or if it is an emergency, gather the bark yourself by pulling it off of the tree by hand. The inner bark is the part used, after the rough, outer bark is removed. The inner bark will tend to come off in strips.

Place the bark in a warm, well-ventilated room and dry it as quickly as possible. Low humidity is a must when drying the bark. Place it on a screen or lay it on a clean wooden floor in the attic. Turn the bark daily, to ensure even drying.

It must be stored in an airtight container to ensure that it does not develop mold or other harmful bacteria. Here's a way to help keep it free from bacteria and mold: Put several drops of camphor (a preservative) on an absorbent cloth. Place the cloth between two sheets of waxed paper and place it in the bottom of the container.

The attic is an ideal place to dry roots and bark, as that room stays warmer and dryer then the rest of the house. I have not been able to dry roots or bark for the last several years because we were in the process of building our home and there was no attic available. A greenhouse is also a great place to dry the roots and barks. I hope my little greenhouse will be built and ready for the early spring. When it is ready, I will use it to dry my roots next fall.

The roots are not to difficult to dry. After digging the roots, wash them thoroughly with a small scrub brush to remove all traces of soil. Drain well and slice the roots crosswise or length-wise. Spread them on a screen in the attic or greenhouse to dry thoroughly. Turn the roots to ensure thorough drying. These roots also need a preservative added to the container. The preservative will ensure that the roots will be protected from insects or mold. Remember, the roots and the bark need to be dried as quickly as possible to ensure a healthy product.

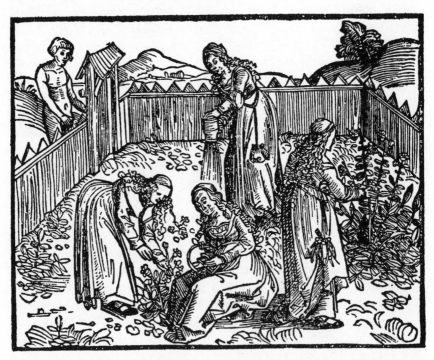

Always date and label the tins or jars in which you store your herbs. In this way, you can keep track of which herbs you have and how fresh they are. The roots can be kept for 3-4 years. The leaves and flowers can be kept for several years, but will probably need to be replaced yearly, because of frequent use. The fleshy roots, such as dandelion and burdock, should be replaced yearly.

I always run out of the herbs that I use to make the infusions because we drink them quite often, for pleasure and for tonic pur-poses. I never know how much to preserve as we use what we have and would probably use a wheelbarrow full if we had it on hand. After a time, you soon know what you use in large quantities and make it a point to preserve more of that. The bee balm and licorice mint, as well as the other mints, seem to get used up pretty fast.

I keep my cooking herbs separate from my medicinal herbs. Some of them overlap, but this is handy, because then I don't run out of any one herb as fast as I might otherwise.

If, during the winter, I find I'm using large quantities of some of the herbs, I plan to plant larger beds of them in the spring. I usually plant more of the herbs that I use regularly for medicine, cooking and beauty preparations. Planning your herb beds and your garden is a wonderful winter past time, a great way to spend your time while waiting for spring. It also helps to make your greenhouse work a little less hectic, as you know exactly what you need to start planting in early spring and can prepare the containers needed. I used to always forget to plant several of the plants that I wanted to grow until I started making my lists ahead of time.

PREPARING YOUR HERBAL MEDICINE CHEST

Now that you have grown, harvested, and dried your herbs—and have a basic knowledge of their many uses—you should prepare your own herbal medicine chest. You do not need a large supply of herbs. Your medicine chest may be designed to hold only a few remedies, but it is important that you have a special place for them. I use a large cabinet in my living room to store all the herbs and herbal preparations. They are handy and ready to use. I take a great deal of pleasure from my cabinet.

As you become more familiar with using the different herbal medicines, you will get some idea of the herbs you will need to keep on hand. Also, your family's habits will determine what you do keep on hand. It's a personal decision; no one can tell you what you need. If someone in the family has a tendency to get chest colds, you would prepare some of those remedies, or at least have on hand different herbs needed to create those remedies so you can treat them at the first sign of illness. Sometimes, by treating a particular illness before it has a chance to get a good hold, we limit the chances of it becoming a serious illness.

By this time, I know what tonics, salves and tinctures we need to keep handy for our family. By keeping some of these on hand we can be prepared for just about any illness or accident. Here is a list of some of the remedies that I keep on hand. I find that I use some frequently and others hardly at all. All of the recipes for these remedies are found in this book, just refer to the chapters that correspond to the illness or disorder mentioned.

1. The menthol camphorated oil is the first thing I would use on any strained muscle, soreness, or arthritis. It's also my first choice for easing chest tightness. The recipe makes a pint, so this lasts me for some time.

2. I like to keep a good assortment of the tinctures on hand. I use the valerian tincture the most. I use it to treat different skin rashes, headaches, and nervousness. I give it to my husband quite often as a way to slow him down so that he gets the rest he needs. If I feel a cold coming on, I use the antibiotic tincture and the rosemary tincture. I usually use calendula to clean cuts and scrapes, but almost any of the tinctures are good for that, so I don't worry too much if I run out of calendula tincture.

3. I always have several of the salves on hand. My husband loves the all-purpose salve and I like to keep that prepared for him. I always keep the balm of Gilead salve ready to treat burns and scratches. My aloe vera grows in several different parts of the house and I always have the fresh leaves handy, so I am not too concerned with making a salve from that. If I had to tend to a more serious burn I would make some.

4. I keep an earache tincture ready for use. I don't get earaches, and neither does my husband, but my grandson does, so I keep it for him. I also use it on my dog, Charley, when he is bothered with ear problems. He is 18 years old now, so I use quite a few of my home remedies to keep him comfortable. He still gets around real well, so the herbs must be of help to him.

5. I always keep the wild cherry cough syrup on hand, and in the fall I try to keep a supply of cough drops. They are delicious. We suck on those even when we don't have a cough.

6. I keep several kinds of herbal capsules prepared for our home use. I make the high blood pressure capsules for my husband, so they are always handy. I take the change of life capsules, along with the capsules for poor circulation. To save time, and to have them ready when I need them, I try to make at least a 2 month supply of the capsules at one time.

7. In the cabinet, I place all the vitamin supplements that we might need to take during bouts of illness. I also stock herbs to make remedies for other, less common needs. The number of herbs that you keep in stock is not as important as your ability to use what you do have.

The dried herbs found in tea or infusion remedies are effective and easy to use, so just keeping them on hand is enough to enable you to treat many personal illnesses. It may take a little time to get the supplies you need, but it is well worth the effort.

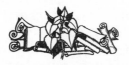

I keep all the cooking herbs in the kitchen spice cabinet. The other herbal preparations designed for bath or personal care are kept in the linen closet or bathroom. The personal care products are used daily and, of course, are kept where they will be at hand.

It really doesn't take as much time as you might think to make the herbs and herbal products for daily use. Even if they did take a lot of time, I still would keep using them for our health's sake. Besides I get a lot of pleasure and enjoyment out of being able to make a lot of the products that are used here at my home. There is a lot of self-satisfaction in using nature's bounty.

SEED AND PLANT SOURCES
In addition to growing my own herbs, I purchase many of the dried herbs and roots from a local health food store, or from mail

order catalogs. There are many that just are not available to me in the wild and I still want to be able to use them.

There are many different sources for herbs. Most of the seed companies carry at least a few herb plants as well as many of the seeds. Your local nurseries will also carry a few. Check with friends and neighbors. You may be surprised at the number of acquaintances that grow a few herbs for their personal use.

I find that most people are more than willing to share starts of plants. I have found that the people who grow herbs are some of the nicest people in the world. They are willing to share stories, remedies, and information along with the herb starts. You can meet some of these wonderful, caring people through garden and herb clubs.

There are many newsletters and magazines that carry information on how to use and where to purchase herbs. This is a never-ending hobby. The more you learn, the more you will want to learn. Many communities are starting herb workshops, homestead groups and classes to help you learn about how to live a more natural lifestyle. If there isn't a class in your neighborhood, perhaps you could start one on canning, soapmaking or other skills that you have. People you meet through any classes that you teach will have other skills that they can teach you. The learning project could grow until there could be many such classes in learning how to live a more natural lifestyle.

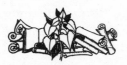

I have listed a few companies here that carry some of the herbs. The first part of the list is devoted to sources for native plants. I feel that it is important that you grow the wild plants in order to become acquainted with their growing habits, as well as to provide an opportunity to learn to identify them.

A few of the companies charge a small fee for their catalogs, but I feel that it is not money wasted. Some handle only the seed for the wild plants, and this is good because it will give you experience in starting your own. If some of the herb seeds are difficult to germinate, just keep in mind that you have to duplicate nature's seasons. Some of the seeds that are not annuals will have to be placed in the refrigerator or freezer for at least a week to duplicate the winter season that these seeds must have in order to germinate.

SOURCES FOR NATIVE PLANTS

Forest Farm
990 Tetherow Road
Williams, OR 97544
(503) 846-6963

"Starter"plants, no wild collected. (This means they grow their own wild plants from wild seed; they do not collect from the wild.) $3.00 for catalog; U.S. sales only.

Johnny's Selected Seeds
310 Foss Hill Road
Albion, Maine 04910
(207) 437-4301

Plants and seeds. Free catalog.

Hayes Regional Arboretum
801 Elks Road
Richmond, IN 47374
(317) 962-3745

Wildflower seed available January through April only. Free seed list.

Missouri Wildflower Nursery
Route 2, Box 373
Jefferson City, MO 65109
(314) 496-3492

Native wildflowers, no wild collected. $2.00 for catalog.

Native Gardens
Route 1, Box 494
Greenback, TN 37742
(615) 856-3350

Native plants, no wild collected. $1.00 for catalog.

Niche Gardens
Route 1 Box 290
Dept. JW
Chapel Hill 27516
(919) 967-0078

Wildflowers, no wild collected. $3.00 for catalog.

Prairie Moon Nursery
Route 3, Box 163
Winona, MN 55987
(507) 452-5231

Native prairie plants and seeds. $2.00 for catalog; $3.00 outside of U.S.

Shady Oaks Nursery
700-19th Avenue N.E.
Waseca, MN 56093
(507)835-5033

Shade garden plants, wildflowers, and ferns. Free catalog; U.S. sales only.

Shooting Star Nursery
311 Bates Road
Frankfort, KY 40601
(502) 223-1679

Native wildflowers, U.S. No wild collected. $1.00 for catalog.

Taylor's Herb Garden, Inc.
1535 Lone Oak Road
Vista, CA 92084
(207) 437-9294

Taylor's carries about 135 different herb plants. $3.00 for catalog; U.S. sales only.

Woodlanders, Inc.
1128 Colleton Avenue
Aiken, SC 29801
(803)648-7522

Native trees, shrubs, and wildflowers. $1.00 for catalog in the U.S.; $2.50 outside of U.S.

WE-DU Nurseries
Route 5, Box 724
Marion, NC 28752
(704) 738-8300

Native and companion plants; no wild collected. $2.00 for catalog.

Wellsweep Herb Farm
317 Mount Bethel Road
Port Murray, NJ 07865
(908) 852-5390

Herb plants and seeds. $2.00 for catalog. U.S. sales only.

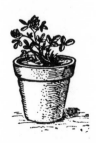

SOURCES FOR DRIED HERBS AND
HERB RELATED PRODUCTS

Frontier Cooperative Herbs
Herb and Spice Collection
Box 299
Norway, IA 52318
(319) 227-7996

This company is a co-op and sells only wholesale. They do offer a catalog for retail sale called "Herb and Spice Collection." Free catalog; U.S. sales only.

Indiana Botanic Gardens, Inc.
P.O. Box 5
Hammond, IN 46325
(219) 947-4040

Dried herbs, spices, and herb related products. Free catalog.

Meadowbrook Herb Garden
93 Kingstown Road
Wyoming, R.I. 02898
(401) 539-7603

Dried herbs, seeds, herb related products. $1.00 for catalog.

Rafal Spice Company
2521 Russell
Detroit, MI 48207
(313) 259-6373

Spices, herb teas, and herb related products. Free catalog.

San Francisco Herb Co.
250-14th Street
Dept. J
San Francisco, CA 94103
California residents: (415) 861-7174
Out-of-state: 1-800-227-4530

Dried herbs, spices, and herb related products. Free catalog.

The Whole Herb Company
250 E. Blithdale Avenue
P.O. Box 1085
Mill Valley, CA 94942
(415) 383-6485

Wholesale only of bulk, dried herbs.

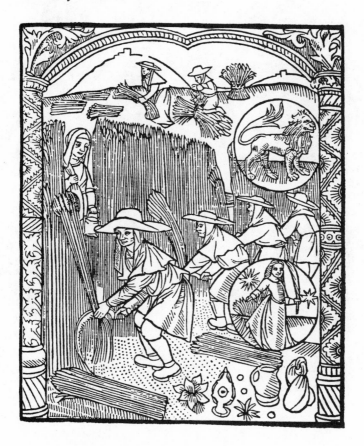

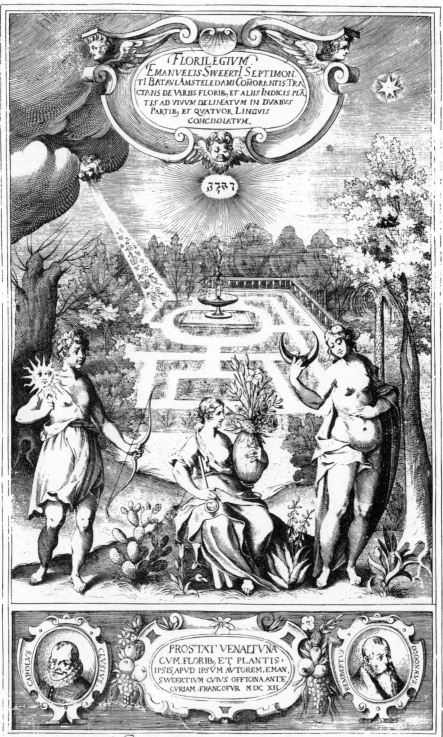

FLORILEGIVM
EMANVELIS SWEERTI SEPTIMON.
TI BATAVI AMSTELEDAMI COMORANTIS, TRA.
CTANS DE VARIIS FLORIB, ET ALIIS INDICIS PLÃ
TIS AD VIVVM DELINEATVM IN DVABVS
PARTIB, ET QVATVOR LINGVIS
CONCINNATVM.

3787

CAROLVS CLVSIVS

PROSTAT VENALI VNA
CVM FLORIB, ET PLANTIS
IPSIS, APVD IPSVM AVTOREM, EMAN.
SWEERTIVM CVIVS OFFICINA ANTE
CVRIAM FRANCOFVR MDC XII.

REMBERTVS DODONÆVS

Impressum Francofurti ad Mœnum Apud Anthonium Kempner sumptib. Autoris. 3 6 12.

Common and Scientific Names of Herbs

ACACIA: *Acacia senegal*
AGRIMONY: *Agrimonia eupatoria*
ALFALFA: *Medicago sativa*
ALKANET: *Alkanna tinctoria*
ALLSPICE: *Lindera benzoin*
ALOE VERA: *Aloe spp.*
ALUM: *L. alumen*
AMARANTH: *Amaranthus hypochondriacus*
ANGELICA: *Angelica archangelica*
ANISE: *Pimpinella anisum*
APPLE: *Pyrus malus*
ARNICA: *Arnica montana*
ARROWROOT: *M. arundinacea*
ASPARAGUS: *Asparagus officinalis*
AVOCADO: *genus Persea*
BALM OF GILEAD: *Populus candicans*
BARBERRY: *Berberis vulgaris*
BARLEY: *Hordeum spp.*
BASIL: *Ocimum basilicum*
BAY: *Laurus nobilis*
BEE BALM: *Monarda didyma*
BEET: *Beta vulgaris*
BETONY: *Stachys officinalis*
BIBLE LEAF: *Chrysanthemum balsamita*
BIRCH: *Betula spp.*
BLACK ALDER: *Prinos verticillatus*
BLACKBERRY: *Rubus species*
BLACK COHOSH: *cimicifuga Racemosa*
BLACK CURRANT: *genus Ribes*
BLACK ELDER: *genus Sambucus*
BLACK MUSTARD: *B. nigra*
BLUEBERRY: *Vaccinium corybosum*

BLUE COHOSH: *Caulophyllum thalictroides*
BLUE VERVAIN: *Verbena hastata*
BONESET: *Eupatorium perfoliatum*
BORAGE: *Borago officinalis*
BROOM: *Cytisus-scoparius*
BRUSSEL SPROUTS: *Brassica oleracea gemmifera*
BUCKTHORN: *Bumelia lycioides*
BURDOCK: *Articum lappa*
CABBAGE: *Brassica species*
CALENDULA: *Calendula officinalis*
CAMPHOR: *Camphor wood*
CANCER ROOT: *Epifagus virginiana*
CARAWAY: *Carum carvi*
CARDAMOM: *Elettaria cardamomum*
CARROT: *Daucus carota*
CASHEW NUT: *Anacardium occidentale*
CASTOR BEAN: *Ricinus communis*
CASTOR OIL: *Ricinus communis*
CATNIP: *Nepeta cataria*
CATTAIL: *Typha latifolia*
CAYENNE PEPPER: *Capsicum annuum*
CELERY: *Apium graveolens*
CHAMOMILE: *Matricaria chamomila, Anthemis nobilis*
CHERRY: *Prunus*
CHERVIL: *Anthriscus cerefolium*
CHICKWEED: *Anagallis arvensis*
CHICORY: *Cichorium intybus*
CHIVES: *Allium schoenoprasum*
CINNAMON: *C. zeylanicum*
CINQUEFOIL: *Popentilla reptans*
CLARY SAGE: *Salvia sclarea*
CLEAVERS: *Galium aparine*
CLEMATIS: *C. virginiana*
CLOVES: *Eugenia aromatica*
COCOA: *Theobroma cacao*
COLTSFOOT: *Tussilago farfara*
COMFREY: *Symphytum officinale*
CORN FLOWERS: *Centauria cyanus*
CORIANDER: *Coriandrum sativum*

COSTMARY: *Chrysanthemum balsamita*
COUGHWORT: *Tussilago farfara*
CRANBERRY: *Vaccinium macrocarpon*
CUCUMBER: *Cucumis sativus*
CUMIN: *Cuminum cyminum*
CURRANTS : *Ribes rubrum*
DANDELION: *Taraxacum officinale*
DILL: *Anethum graveolens*
DOCK: *Rumex spp.*
ECHINACEA: *Echinacea angustifolia*
ELDERBERRY: *Sambucus nigra, S. canadensis*
ELDER: *Sambucus canadensis*
ELECAMPANE: *Inula helenium*
EUCALYPTUS: *Eucalyptus globulus*
EYEBRIGHT: *Euphrasia officinalis*
FENNEL: *Foeniculum vulgare*
FENUGREEK: *Trigonella foenum-graecum*
FEVERFEW: *Chrysanthemum parthenium*
FLAX SEED: *Linum usitatissimum*
FOXGLOVE: *Digitalis purpurea*
GALL: *Quercus infectoria*
GARLIC: *Allium sativum*
GENTIAN: *Gentiania lutea*
GERANIUM: *Geranium maculatum*
GERMANDER: *Teucrium chamaedrys*
GINGER: *Zingiber officinale*
GINSENG: *Panax quinquefolius*
GOLDTHREAD: *Coptis greenlandica*
GOLDENROD: *Solidago*
GOLDENSEAL: *Hydrastis canadensis*
GREEN BEANS: *genus Phaseolus*
GREEN ELDER: *genus Sambucus*
GREEN PEPPER: *C. grossium*
GOURD SEED: *Cucurbitaceae*
HAWTHORN: *Crataegus oxyacantha*
HEARTSEASE: *Viola tricolor*
HEDGE APPLE: *Maclura pomifera*
HENNA: *Lawsonia alba, L. inermis*
HOLY THISTLE: *Cnicus benedictus*

HOLLYHOCKS: *Althea rosea*
HONEYSUCKLE: *Diervilla lonicera*
HOPS: *Humulus lupulus*
HOREHOUND: *Marrubium vulgare*
HORSERADISH: *Armoracia rusticana*
HORSETAIL: *Equisetum hyemale*
HYSSOP: *Hyssopus officinalis*
IRISH MOSS: *Chondrus crispus, Gigartina mamillosa*
IVY: *Hedera helix*
JEWELWEED: *Impatiens biflora*
JOB'S TEARS: *Coiz lacryma Jobi*
JUNIPER BERRIES: *Juniperus communis*
KELP: *Fucus vesiculosis*
KIDNEY BEANS: *Phaseolus vulgaris*
LAVENDER: *Lavandula angustifolia*
LEMON: *Citrus limon*
LEMON BALM: *Melissa officinalis*
LEMON THYME: *T. serpyllum*
LEMON VERBENA: *Aloysia triphylla*
LETTUCE: *Lactuca sativa*
LICORICE: *Glycyrrhiza glabra*
LIME BLOSSOMS: *Tilia europea, T. americana*
LINDEN: *Tilia europea, T. americana*
LINSEED: *Linum usitatissimum*
LOBELIA: *Lobelia inflata*
LUFFA: *L. aegyptiaca*
LOVAGE: *Levisticum officinale*
MEADOW SWEET: *Spirea Ulmaria*
MALE FERN: *Dryopteris filix-mas*
MALLOW: *Malva rotundifolia*
MARSH MALLOW: *Althaea officinalis*
MARJORAM: *Origanum majorana*
MAY APPLE: *Podophyllum peltatum*
MEXICAN MARIGOLD: *genus Tagetes*
MILKTHISTLE: *Lactuca scariola L.*
MILK WEED: *Asclepias*
MINTS: *Mentha spp.*
MOTHERWORT: *Leonorus cardiaca*
MUGWORT: *Artemisia vulgaris*

MULLEIN: *Verbascum thapsus*
MUSTARD: *Brassica, various species*
MULBERRIES: *Morus nigra*
MYRRH: *C. Myrrha*
NASTURTIUM: *Tropaeolum majus*
NETTLE: *Urtica dioica*
NEW JERSEY TEA: *Ceanot americanus*
NUTMEG: *Myristica fragrans*
OAK: *Quercus varieties*
OKRA: *Hibiscus esculentus*
ONION: *Allium cepa*
ORANGE: *C. Sinensis*
ORANGE BLOSSOMS: *C. Sinensis*
OREGANO: *Origanum vulgare*
ORRIS ROOT: *Florentine iris*
PANSY: *Viola tricolor*
PAPAYA: *Carica papaya*
PARSLEY: *Petroselinum crispum*
PASSION FLOWER: *Passiflora incarnata*
PEACH LEAVES: *Amygdalus persica*
PEA: *Pisum sativum*
PEAR: *Pyrus communis*
PENNYROYAL: *Mentha pulegium*
PEPPERGRASS: *Lepidium virginicum*
PEPPERMINT: *Mentha piperita*
PILEWORT: *Amaranthus cruenyus*
PINEAPPLE: *Ananas comosus*
PLANTAIN: *Plantago major*
PLEURISY ROOT: *Asclepias tuberosa*
POKEWEED: *Phytolacca decandra*
POMEGRANATE: *Punica granatum*
POPLAR: *Populus spp. salicaceae*
POTATO: *Solanum tuberosum*
POT MARIGOLD: *Calendula officinalis*
POWDERED SUGAR
PRICKLY LETTUCE: *Lactuca virosa, L. scariola*
PRIMROSE: *Primula*
PRUNES: *Prunum*
PSYLLIUM SEED: *Plantage psyllium*

PUFFBALL MUSHROOM: *Lycoperdon*
PUMPKIN SEED: *Cucurbita pepo*
PURSLANE: *Portulaca oleracea*
QUEEN ANNE'S LACE: *Daucus carota*
RAGWEED: *Ambrosia artemesiaefolia*
RASPBERRY: *Rubus idaeus*
RED CEDAR: *Juniperus virginiana*
RED CLOVER: *Trifolium pratense*
RED OAK BARK: *Quercus varieties*
RICE: *Zizania aquatica*
ROSE: *Rosa spp.*
ROSEHIPS: *Rosagallica, R. canina*
ROSEMARY: *Rosmarinus officinalis*
RUBBING ALCOHOL
RUE: *Ruta graveolens*
SAFFLOWER OIL: *Cathamus tinctorius*
SAGE: *Salvia officinalis*
SARSAPARILLAS: *Aralia nudicaulis*
SASSAFRAS: *Sassafras albidum*
SAVORY: *Satureja spp.*
SAFFRON: *Crocus sativus*
SHEEP SORREL: *Rumex acetosella*
SHEPHERDS PURSE: *Capsella bursa-pastoris*
SEPTFOIL: *Potentilla tormentilla*
SILVER BIRCH: *Betula alleghaniensis*
SLIPPERY ELM: *Ulmus fulvus*
SOAPWEED: *Yucca filamentosa*
SOAPWORT: *Saponaria officinalis*
SOLOMON'S SEAL: *Polygonatum officinale*
SOYA POWDER
SPEARMINT: *Mentha spicata*
SPINACH: *Spinacia oleracea*
SQUASH: *Cucurbita*
ST. JOHN'S WORT: *Hypericum perforatum*
STRAWBERRY: *Wild, Fragaria virginiana, Garden, Fragaria vesca*
SUNFLOWER: *Helianthus annus*
SWEET CICELY: *Myrrhis odorata*
SWEET FERN: *Myrica asplenifolia*
SWEET WILLIAM: *Saponaria officinalis*

SWEET WOODRUFF: *Galium odoratum*
TOBACCO: *Nicotiana tabacum*
TAG ELDER: *Alnus serrulata*
TANSY: *Tanacetum vulgare*
TARRAGON: *Artemisia dracunculus*
THROATWORT: *Campanula trachelium*
THYME: *Thymus vulgaris*
TOMATO: *Lycopersicon esulentum*
TURNIP: *Brassica Napoprassica*
VALERIAN: *Polemonium caeruleum*
VANILLA: *Vanilla planifolia*
VERBENA: *Verbena urticaefolia L.*
VIOLET: *Viola odorata*
WALNUT: *White walnut, Juglans Cinera; Black walnut, uglans nigra; European walnut, Juglans regia*
WATERCRESS: *Nasturtium officinale*
WATERMELON: *Citrullus vulgaris*
WHITE OAK: *Quercus stellata*
WILD CHERRY: *Prunus serotina*
WILD YAM: *Dioscorea villosa*
WILLOW: *Salix spp.*
WINTERGREEN: *Gaultheria procumbens*
WITCH HAZEL: *Hamamelis virginiana*
WOAD: *Genista tinctoria*
WORMWOOD: *Artemisia absinthium*
YARROW: *Achillea millefolium*
YERBA SANTA: *Eriodictyon californicum, E. glutinosum*
YUCCA ROOT: *Yucca filamentosa*

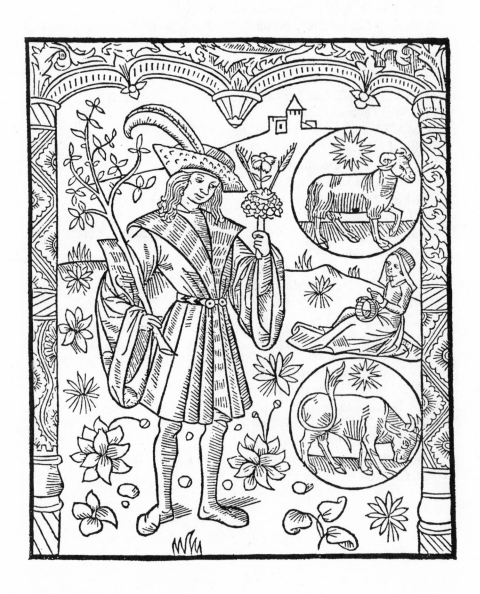

Glossary

ACNE: An inflammatory disease of the sebaceous glands and hair follicles of the skin.

ALIMENTARY CANAL OR TRACT: The digestive tube from the mouth to the anus, including the mouth, pharynx, esophagus, stomach, large and small intestines, and rectum.

ALTERATIVE: Helps to alter or correct minor functional disorders of the system. Also called a blood purifier.

ANEMIA: A condition in which the blood is deficient in red blood cells or in hemoglobin.

ANHYDROUS: Lacking water.

ANTIBIOTIC: Natural substance that inhibits growth or destroys micro-organisms. Used to treat infectious diseases.

ANTISEPTIC: Substance that checks the growth or action of micro-organisms.

APHRODISIAC: Excites sexual desire.

AROMATIC: Has an agreeable odor, and has slightly stimulative action or properties.

ARTHRITIS: Inflammation of a joint, accompanied by pain and swelling.

ASTRINGENT: An agent that has a binding or constricting effect, i.e., one that checks hemorrhages or secretions by coagulation of proteins on a cell surface.

BLOOD PURIFIER: See alterative.

BRONCHITIS: Inflammation of the mucous membrane of the bronchial system.

CANKER: An ulcerous sore on the lips, cheek or tongue.

CARMINATIVE: Expels gas from the stomach, bowels and intestines.

CATARRH: Simple inflammation of the mucous membrane in the respiratory tract.

COLIC: Cramping of the stomach or intestines.

CYSTITIS: Inflammation of the bladder.

DECOCTION: The liquid left after boiling the herb root or bark to extract the properties.

DEMULCENT: Soothing properties in specific herbs that allay the action of stimulating or overacting herbs. Soothing to irritated mucous membranes.

DIAPHORETIC: Increases perspiration. Aids in removing toxins and wastes through the skin.

DIURETIC: Increases the flow of urine and aids in elimination of waste products and toxins through the urine.

DROPSY: An accumulation of excess water and fluid in the subcutaneous tissues or cavities of the body.

ECZEMA: Acute or chronic inflammatory condition of the skin. May manifest as crusts, scales or pustules—alone or in combination. More of a symptom than a disease.

EMOLLIENT: Use externally and internally for a soothing or healing effect.

ENZYMES: Complex proteins that are capable of inducing chemical changes in other substances without being changed themselves.

EPIDERMAL: Outer layer of skin.

EXCRETIONS: Waste matter. The elimination of waste products from the body.

EXPECTORANT: Facilitates the expulsion of mucus from the respiratory tract.

EXUDATION: Oozing of fluids or accumulation of fluid in a cavity.

FLATULENCE: Excessive gas in the alimentary canal.

GASTRITIS: Inflammation of the stomach lining.

GERMICIDAL: Any agent which destroys germs or micro-organisms.

GRAVEL: The formation of small concretions in the urinary passages.

HEPATITIS: Inflammation of the liver.

INFUSION: The process of steeping herbs in boiling or hot water to extract the properties of the herb. Used as a tea.

LAXATIVE: Corrects constipation by increasing bowel movements.

MUCILAGINOUS: Gummy or sticky substance that is soothing to areas that are inflamed.

MUCOUS: Having the nature of or resembling mucus.

MUCOUS MEMBRANE: Membrane lining passages and cavities communicating with the air.

NERVINE: Treatment for the nervous system. Quiets nervous irritation due to excitement, fatigue, grief, or headaches.

PLEURISY: Inflammation of the membranes that envelope the lungs and thorax.

POULTICE: Herbs that are finely ground and then moistened, and applied to affected area.

PSORIASIS: Chronic, genetically determined lesions of the skin.

RELAXANT: Substance that relieves stress, strain and tension.

RHEUMATISM: Painful inflammation and swelling of muscles and joints.

SEDATIVE: Soothes nervous excitement and has a quieting effect upon the nervous system without having a narcotic effect.

SPASM: Involuntary contraction of a muscle or a muscle fiber.

STEEP: To extract the essence of by soaking.

STIMULANT: Increases functional actions of the body.

TONIC: Restores strength to the whole system and helps different organs.

UTERINE: Relates to the uterus or the womb.

Bibliography

The Audubon Society Field Guide to North American Wildflowers: Eastern Region. Chanticleer Press Edition. New York: Alfred A. Knopf, 1979.

Crockett, James Underwood and Tanner, Ogden. *The Time-Life Encyclopedia of Gardening Herbs.* Alexandria, VA: Time-Life Books, 1977.

Faelten, Sharon *The Allergy Self-Help Book.* Emmaus, PA: Rodale Press, 1983.

Harrop, Renny, ed. *Encyclopedia of Herbs.* Secaucus, NJ: Chartwell Books, 1977.

Hendler, Dr. Sheldon Saul. *The Doctors' Vitamin and Mineral Encyclopedia.* New York: Simon and Schuster, 1990.

Hermann, Matthias. *Herbs and Medicinal Flowers.* Galahad Books, 1973.

Kresanek, Dr. Jaraslav. *Healing Plants.* Handbook Guide. New York: Arco Publishing, 1985.

Kowalchik, Claire and Hylton, William. *Rodale's Illustrated Encyclopedia of Herbs.* Emmaus, PA: Rodale Press, 1983.

Taber's Cyclopedic Medical Dictionary. Philadelphia: F.A. Davis Company, 1985.

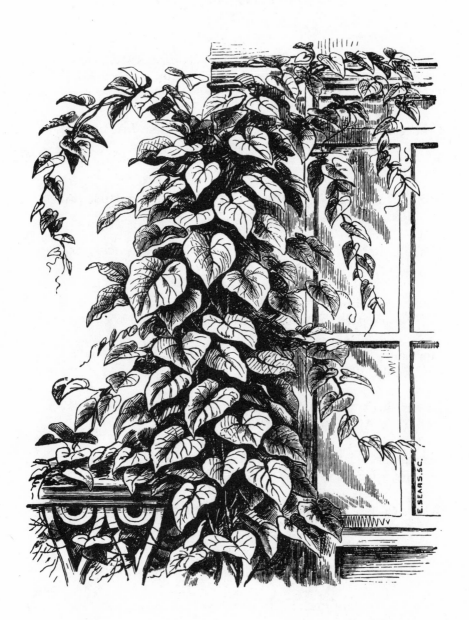

INDEX

STAY IN TOUCH

On the following pages you will find listed, with their current prices, some of the books now available on related subjects. Your book dealer stocks most of these and will stock new titles in the Llewellyn series as they become available. We urge your patronage.

To obtain our full catalog, to keep informed about new titles as they are released and to benefit from informative articles and helpful news, you are invited to write for our bimonthly news magazine/catalog, *Llewellyn's New Worlds of Mind and Spirit*. A sample copy is free, and it will continue coming to you at no cost as long as you are an active mail customer. Or you may subscribe for just $7.00 in U.S.A. and Canada ($20.00 overseas, first class mail). Many bookstores also have *New Worlds* available to their customers. Ask for it.

Stay in touch! In *New Worlds'* pages you will find news and features about new books, tapes and services, announcements of meetings and seminars, articles helpful to our readers, news of authors, products and services, special money-making opportunities, and much more.

Llewellyn's New Worlds of Mind and Spirit
P.O. Box 64383-869, St. Paul, MN 55164-0383, U.S.A.
* * *

TO ORDER BOOKS AND TAPES

If your book dealer does not have the books described on the following pages readily available, you may order them directly from the publisher by sending full price in U.S. funds, plus $3.00 for postage and handling for orders *under* $10.00; $4.00 for orders *over* $10.00. There are no postage and handling charges for orders over $50.00. Postage and handling rates are subject to change. UPS Delivery: We ship UPS whenever possible. Delivery guaranteed. Provide your street address as UPS does not deliver to P.O. Boxes. UPS to Canada requires a $50.00 minimum order. Allow 4-6 weeks for delivery. Orders outside the U.S.A. and Canada: Air-mail—add retail price of book; add $5.00 for each non-book item (tapes, etc.); add $1.00 per item for surface mail.

FOR GROUP STUDY AND PURCHASE

Because there is a great deal of interest in group discussion and study of the subject matter of this book, we feel that we should encourage the adoption and use of this particular book by such groups by offering a special quantity price to group leaders or agents.

Our Special Quantity Price for a minimum order of five copies of *Jude's Herbal Home Remedies* is $29.85 cash-with-order. This price includes postage and handling within the United States. Minnesota residents must add 6.5% sales tax. For additional quantities, please order in multiples of five. For Canadian and foreign orders, add postage and handling charges as above. Credit card (VISA, Master-Card, American Express) orders are accepted. Charge card orders only ($15.00 minimum order) may be phoned in free within the U.S.A. or Canada by dialing 1-800-THE-MOON. For customer service, call 1-612-291-1970. Mail orders to:

LLEWELLYN PUBLICATIONS
P.O. Box 64383-869, St. Paul, MN 55164-0383, U.S.A.

CUNNINGHAM'S ENCYCLOPEDIA OF MAGICAL HERBS
by Scott Cunningham

This is an expansion on the material presented in his first Llewellyn book, *Magical Herbalism*. This is not just another herbal for medicinal uses of herbs—this is the most comprehensive source of herbal data for magical uses ever printed! Almost every one of the over 400 herbs are illustrated, making this a great source for herb identification. For each herb you will also find: magical properties, planetary rulerships, genders, associated deities, folk and Latin names and much more. To make this book even easier to use you will also find a folk name cross reference, and all of the herbs are fully indexed. There is also a large annotated bibliography, and a list of mail order suppliers so you can find the books and herbs you need.

Like all of Scott's books, this one does not require you to use complicated rituals or expensive magical paraphernalia. Instead, it shares with you the intrinsic powers of the herbs. Thus, you will be able to discover which herbs, by their very nature, can be used for luck, love, success, money, divination, astral projection, safety, psychic self-defense and much more. Besides being interesting and educational it is also fun, and fully illustrated with unusual woodcuts from old herbals. This book has rapidly become the classic in its field.

0-87542-122-9, 352 pgs., 6 x 9, illus., softcover $12.95

MAGICAL AROMATHERAPY: THE POWER OF SCENT
by Scott Cunningham

Scent magic has a rich, colorful history. Today, in the shadow of the next century, there is much we can learn from the simple plants that grace our planet. Most have been used for countless centuries. The energies still vibrate within their aromas.

Scott Cunningham, author of *The Complete Book of Incense, Oils and Brews*, has now combined the current knowledge of the physiological and psychological effects of natural fragrances with the ancient art of magical perfumery. In writing this book, he drew on extensive experimentation and observation, research into 4,000 years of written records, and the wisdom of respected aromatherapy practitioners.

Magical Aromatherapy contains a wealth of practical tables of aromas of the seasons, days of the week, the planets, and zodiac; use of essential oils with crystals; synthetic and genuine oils and hazardous essential oils. It also contains a handy appendix of aromatherapy organizations and distributors of essential oils and dried plant products.

0-87542-129-6, 224 pgs., mass market, illus. $3.95

FULL CIRCLE: A SONG OF ECOLOGY
and EARTHEN SPIRITUALITY
Lone Wolf Circles, Forewords by Barbara Mor and Bill Devall

It is common knowledge that we are in a severe ecological crisis. But knowledge of our global predicament is not enough. According to author Lone Wolf Circles, the solution lies in a deep, personal, visceral and spiritual reaction. Full Circle serves as a catalyst for that reaction. It is lyric essay, visionary art and poetry, combined as tools of the sorcerer, inviting personal transformation and invoking crucial planetary change. It is a song, a ritual chant that helps us in the urgent return to our wild, expanded selves.

In the tradition of Gray Snyder, Starhawk and Joseph Campbell, Lone Wolf's art and writings invite, incite and invoke. More a howl than an academic lecture, Full Circle unleashes the spirits of an endangered planet to roam the corridors of our wildest imagination.

0-87542-347-7, 192 pgs., 9" x 8", original artwork, softcover $12.95

THE GAIA TRADITION
by Kisma Stepanich

The Gaia Tradition provides a spiritual foundation upon which women, from all walks of life, can find support and direction. It is an eclectic blend of Wicca, Native American Spirituality and Dianic Goddess worship. Ms. Stepanich guides the reader to spiritual attunement to Mother Earth—through the evolution of the Goddess within, and through connection to the Goddess without.

This book describes the Goddess philosophy and takes us month by month, season by season, through magical celebrations of the Goddess. It includes valuable information for the avid ritualist/ceremonialist and lists 2,000 names and origins of the Goddess from diverse cultures.

Through a series of lessons that deal with beliefs, deep ecology, rituals, spells and more, *The Gaia Tradition* helps women take a more dignified stance in their everyday lives and begin to walk the path of a whole and self-assured person.

0-87542-766-9, 304 pgs., 6 x 9, illustrations, photos, bibliography, index, softcover $12.95

THE COMPLETE HANDBOOK OF NATURAL HEALING
Marcia Starck

Got an itch that won't go away? Want a massage but don't know the difference between Rolfing, Reichian Therapy and Reflexology? Tired of going to the family doctor for minor illnesses that you know you could treat at home—if you just knew how?

Designed to function as a home reference guide, (yet enjoyable and interesting enough to be read straight through), this book addresses all natural healing modalities in use today: dietary regimes, nutritional supplements, cleansing and detoxification, vitamins and minerals, herbology, homeopathic medicine and cell salts, traditional Chinese medicine, Ayurvedic medicine, body work therapies, exercise, mental and spiritual therapies, and more. In addition, a section of 41 specific ailments outlines natural treatments for everything from acne to varicose veins.

0-87542-742-1, 416 pgs., 6 x 9 , diagrams, appendices, bibliography, index, soft-cover **$12.95**

RECLAIMING WOMAN'S VOICE: BECOMING WHOLE
Lesley Shore, Ph.D.

Many of today's difficulties stem from a fundamental imbalance in the core of our world. We have lost our ties with mother Earth and the feminine in our nature. The feminine is suppressed, oppressed — abused. And while everyone suffers the consequences of society's devaluation of the feminine, this book primarily explores its effects on women.

Women's voice finds expression in psychological and psychosomatic symptoms. Many women are depressed or anxious. They are troubled by low self-esteem and suffer from eating disorders and other addictions. They question their beauty and their bodies.

This book shows women how to discover what their symptoms are telling them about their hidden needs and blocked energies. Once the cause of these symptoms are found, women can then move on with their lives, become whole human beings, live in harmony with inner rhythms, and finally feel good about themselves.

0-87542-722-7, 208 pgs., 5-1/4 x 8 , softcover **$9.95**

EARTH MOTHER ASTROLOGY
by Marcia Starck

Now, for the first time, a book that combines the science of astrology with the current interest in crystals, herbs, aromas, and holistic health. With this book and a copy of your astrological birth chart (readily available from sources listed in the book) you can use your horoscope to benefit your total being—body, mind and spirit. Learn, for example, what special nutrients you need during specific planetary cycles, or what sounds or colors will help you transform emotional states during certain times of the year.

This is a compendium of information for those interested in health and astrology. For the beginner, it explains all the astrological signs, planets and houses in a simple and yet new way, physiologically as well as symbolically.

This is a book of modern alchemy, showing the reader how to work with earth energies to achieve healing and transformation, thereby creating a sense of the cosmic unity of all Earth's elements.

0-87542-741-3, 288 pgs., 5-1/4 x 8, illus., softcover $12.95

IN THE SHADOW OF THE SHAMAN
by Amber Wolfe

Presented in what the author calls a "cookbook shamanism" style, this book shares recipes, ingredients, and methods of preparation for experiencing some very ancient wisdoms—wisdoms of Native American and Wiccan traditions, as well as contributions from other philosophies of Nature, as they are used in the shamanic way. Wolfe encourages us to feel confident and free to use her methods to cook up something new, completely on our own. This blending of ancient formulas and personal methods represents what Ms. Wolfe calls "Aquarian Shamanism."

In the Shadow of the Shaman is designed to communicate in the most practical, direct ways possible, so that the wisdom and the energy may be shared for the benefits of all. Whatever your system or tradition, you will find this to be a valuable book, a resource, a friend, a gentle guide and support on your journey. Dancing in the shadow of the shaman, you will find new dimensions of Spirit.

0-87542-888-6, 384 pgs., 6 x 9, illus., softcover $12.95

THE LLEWELLYN ANNUALS

ALL NEW! **Llewellyn's LUNAR ORGANIC GARDENER:** For the past 90 years, thousands of Llewellyn's *Moon Sign Book* users have testified to the amazing powers of lunar gardening. Now Llewellyn's *Lunar Organic Gardener* brings together the best of ancient lunar methods with time-tested and leading-edge organic techniques to give you exciting alternative approaches to your growing endeavors. Dedicated experts in the field contribute articles on practical ways in which you can work harmoniously with nature. Plus, everything you need to plan your own lunar organic garden or crops is provided in the handy tables. Discover the spiritual side to gardening, and marvel at your results. **$3.95**

Llewellyn's MOON SIGN BOOK: Approximately 400 pages of valuable information on gardening, fishing, weather, stock market forecasts, personal horoscopes, good planting dates, and general instructions for finding the best date to do just about anything! Articles by prominent forecasters and writers in the fields of gardening, astrology, politics, economics and cycles. This special almanac, different from any other, has been published annually since 1906. It's fun, informative and has been a great help to millions in their daily planning. **State year $4.95**

Llewellyn's SUN SIGN BOOK: Your personal horoscope for the entire year! All 12 signs are included in one handy book. Also included are forecasts, special feature articles, and an action guide for each sign. Monthly horoscopes for your personal Sun Sign are written by Gloria Star, author of *Optimum Child*. And, there are articles on a variety of subjects written by well-known astrologers from around the country. Much more than just a horoscope guide! Entertaining and fun all year. **State year $4.95**

Llewellyn's ASTROLOGICAL CALENDAR: Large wall calendar of 48 pages. Beautiful full-color cover and full color inside. Includes special feature articles by famous astrologers, and complete introductory information on astrology. It also contains a lunar gardening guide, celestial phenomena, a blank horoscope chart, and monthly date pages which include aspects, Moon phases, signs and voids, planetary motion, an ephemeris, personal forecasts, lucky dates, planting and fishing dates, and more. The size is 10" x 13." Set in Central time, with fold-down conversion table for other time zones worldwide. **State year $9.95**

TREATING FOOD ALLERGY MY WAY
Exploring the Most Important Food Allergies
by William E. Walsh, M.D.

Do you or does someone you know suffer from migraine headaches with no apparent cause? Have you ever had spells of fatigue or inability to concentrate? These problems may not be in your head . . . they may be in your diet!

Years of medical practice have taught Dr. Walsh that many common foods and beverages force his patients to suffer uncomfortable and painful symptoms: fatigue, diarrhea, rashes, hyperactivity, canker sores, irritability, joint aches and more. In *Treating Food Allergy My Way,* he talks about the illnesses that affect his patients and describes a diet and lifestyle plan that helps reduce these irritating and uncomfortable symptoms.

Dr. Walsh presents an overview of food allergy and the biochemical processes involved in clear, simple language. He then discusses the most common food allergens including citrus, MSG, refined sugar, corn, artificial sweeteners and much, much more. Learn how to read food labels for harmful additives and chemicals, and find out what is safe to order when dining out. Includes 47 easily tolerated recipes.

0-9631544-3-5, 176 pgs., 6 x 9, bibliography $9.95

THE JOY OF HEALTH
A Doctor's Guide to Nutrition and Alternative Medicine
by Zoltan P. Rona M.D., M.Sc.

Finally, a medical doctor objectively explores the benefits and pitfalls of alternative health care, based on exceptional nutritional scholarship, long clinical practice, and wide-ranging interactions with "established" and alternative practitioners throughout North America.

The Joy of Health is must reading before you seek the advice of an alternative health care provider. Can a chiropractor or naturopath help your condition? What are viable alternatives to standard cancer care? Is Candida a real disease? Can you really extend your life with megavitamins? Might hidden food allergies be the root of many physical and emotional problems?

- Get clear-cut answers to the most commonly asked questions about nutrition and preventive medicine
- Explore various treatments for 47 conditions and diseases
- Make informed choices about food, diets and supplements
- Discover startling information about food allergies and related conditions
- Explore 20 different types of diets and recipes
- Cut through advertising claims and vested-interest scare tactics
- Empower yourself to achieve a high level of wellness

0-87542-684-0, 264 pgs., 6 x 9, softcover $12.95